A Community of One

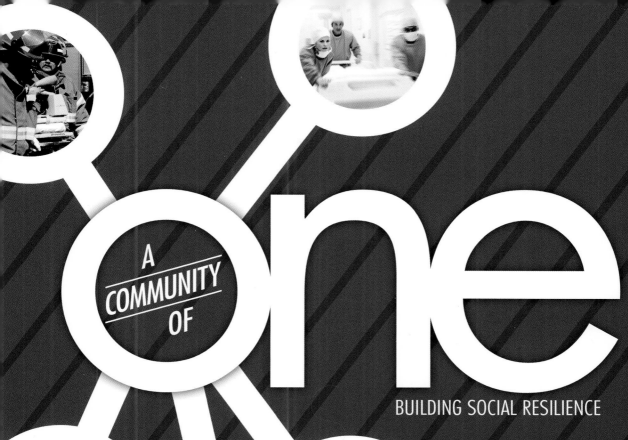

A COMMUNITY OF one

BUILDING SOCIAL RESILIENCE

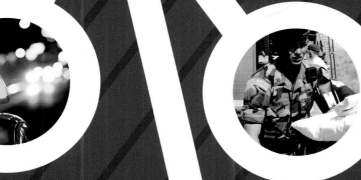

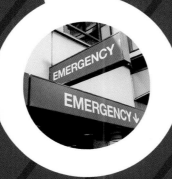

MICHAEL WM. MARKS

PHIL CALLAHAN

MIKE GRILL

Copyright © 2019 by
PennWell Corporation
1421 South Sheridan Road
Tulsa, Oklahoma 74112-6600 USA

800.752.9764
+1.918.831.9421
sales@pennwell.com
www.FireEngineeringBooks.com

Managing Editor: Mark Haugh
Production Manager: Tony Quinn
Cover Designer: Beth Rose
Book Designer: Susan E. Ormston

Library of Congress Cataloging-in-Publication Data
Names: Marks, Michael Wm., 1946- author. | Callahan, Phil, author. | Grill, Michael, author.
Title: A community of one : building social resilience / Michael Wm. Marks, Phil Callahan, Mike Grill.
Description: Tulsa, Oklahoma : PennWell Corporation, [2018] | Includes bibliographical references and index.
Identifiers: LCCN 2018023210 | ISBN 9781593704568
Subjects: LCSH: Resilience (Personality trait) | First responders—Job stress. | Emergency medical personnel--Job stress. | Stress management.
Classification: LCC BF698.35.R47 M36 2018 | DDC 158.7--dc23

Printed in the United States of America

1 2 3 4 5   23 22 21 20 19

Aspen groves

Mother Nature's reminder

That while there are

Wondrous individual trees

They are all held together by a common root.

— MM

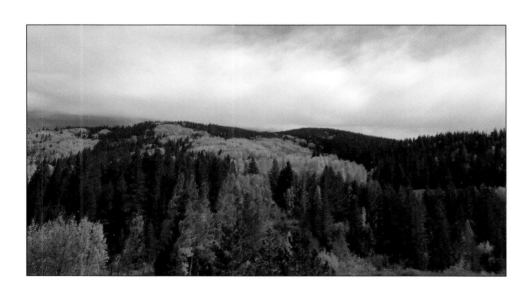

CONTENTS

ACKNOWLEDGMENTS

Alone we can do so little; together we can do so much.

— Helen Keller

After more than a decade of working with student veterans, first responders, and health care providers, there are far too many people to thank for their input, insights, and ideas. All have been driven by a desire to be of service to a vision greater than themselves. They have held to the belief that by learning these skills, they and others can improve the quality of their personal and professional lives.

Neil Atkinson, PE, and his editorial skills have been invaluable to this project going back nearly to its origins. He, among all of us at One Tree Learning Institute (www.onetreelearning. org), has embraced our vision with the most enthusiasm. Without his diligence, this work would not be possible.

There are, of course, the *early adapters* who inspired and encouraged this work. Dr. Terri Riffe, Dr. Kris Weatherly, Dr. Erin Doktor, the staff of the University of Arizona Teaching Center and College of Agriculture, Jim Shockey, PhD, dean of the University of Arizona South, and Alice Packard, LCSW, at the Southern Arizona VA Health Care System saw the importance of this work and its value to the student veteran community.

Dale Crogan and Tony Lo Giudice of the Mesa Fire and EMS community were the first to see the benefits of this work to the first responder community. It is because of their foresight that this curriculum is now part of the Mesa Fire and Police Training Academy. Seeing the success of this program, they have been strong advocates of providing first responders with the psychological and behavioral skills to cope with the demands of their work. Having dealt firsthand with the loss of responders to PTSD, burnout, and suicide, these two men have dedicated themselves to making sure that first responders have the mental armor they need to have long, productive careers.

Mike Grill, Jeff Dyar, and Jonathan Gunderson have been critical in circulating this work both nationally and in Colorado's first responder community.

Dr. Wanda Larson and the Resilience Team at the University of Arizona College of Nursing have been a gift. Heidi Kosanke, Lindsay Bouchard, Patricia Wilger, and Christine Pasquet have inspired us to find the most effective ways to disseminate this course to aspiring nurses. Their passion to assist young nurses to have long and meaningful careers has fueled this work.

To say thank you, while a small token, is most heartfelt.

INTRODUCTION

*The two most important days in your life are the day you are born
and the day you find out why.*

— Mark Twain

WHY THIS BOOK

Simon Sinek, in his TED talk "Start with Why," artfully explained that when we understand *why* we are doing something, *why* we feel passionate about it, and *why* it gives us meaning, the *how* and *what* emerge. The *why* of this book is complex and not given to an easy sound bite. It is an outgrowth of work begun by Dr. Phil Callahan and Dr. Michael William Marks working with student veterans transitioning from the military to college life. We both grew up with fathers from the Greatest Generation (WWII), where a sense of service was a core value, not a punch line. Dr. Callahan became an educator and academic, with a passion for innovative curricula and better ways to engage students in learning. Along the way, as a result of his Eagle Scout training and his need to be of service, he became a volunteer firefighter and EMT-P in rural southwestern Arizona, all while teaching at the University of Arizona South, in Sierra Vista.

My *why* is the result of more than 40 years of treating survivors of trauma, whether civilian or military. For me, the answer came into focus one afternoon in 2005, when I was team leader of the post-traumatic stress disorder (PTSD) outpatient clinic at the Southern Arizona VA Health Care System. That afternoon I saw three young Operation Enduring Freedom/ Operation Iraqi Freedom veterans who had been honorably discharged from the military and who shared aspirations of attending college. Independently, each had the same story of struggles with concentration and memory, hyperarousal, anger, and frustration.

> *Steve was an intense man of Hispanic descent, with a curiosity about the why of the world. He had been in the Army's 82nd Airborne and completed two tours in Afghanistan. His dream was to be the first in his family to attend college. He summed up the tone of all three young men when he said, "Those kids' minds are like sponges; they soak up everything. I'm lucky to remember my name some days. Then they had no respect for the instructor, questioning everything, which just made me pissed off at them and the professor. I started avoiding class and eventually dropped out."*

> *As each one told their story, the faces of Vietnam veterans who had shared the same story some 30 years earlier swept through my mind. And with each telling an old rage grew in me so that by the end of the day I had made a promise to myself, "I'll be damned if I'm going to let this happen again to another generation of veterans. Not on my watch!"*

Thus began the journey that led to this book.

The first step began with the creation of the Supportive Education for Returning Veterans (SERV) curriculum, which consisted of a resilience course, a teaching-to-learn course, and a course on leadership.[1] It was a cohort, learner-centered, problem-based curriculum that remains the foundation of this work. Work in the field of resilience and academic success clearly shows that resiliency scores are a better predictor of the probability of a student staying in college and graduating. It is better a forecaster than SAT scores, high school GPA, or ranking in high school.[2,3,4] Our work with student veterans, most of whom had PTSD or traumatic brain injury (TBI) or both, showed statistically significant increases in their resilience scores from the beginning of the semester to the end. In fact, 90% of the two pilot groups stayed in school and graduated.[5] Even more satisfying was the fact that many went on to graduate with advanced degrees.

Eventually, the resiliency course found its way into the first responder community, where these heroes are exposed to the same types of situations, on a daily basis, that veterans often endure.[6,7,8] Tragically, both veterans and first responders have suicide rates that exceed the general population.[9,10,11] In fact, among occupational groupings, workplace suicide was highest among the protective services personnel (e.g., police and firefighters), with medical providers ranking third.[12,13] For me, these staggering statistics are part of the *why* that demanded this book. Everyone who has participated in creating this book has their own *why* they have a passion about this work. As if to underscore the importance of this book, a dear friend who is a former Navy SEAL and Vietnam veteran is fond of saying, "We are all veterans of something."

The results of this work have been promising, with first responders having statistically significant increases in their resilience scores as a result of the training. This is gratifyingly similar to our results with veterans.[14,15,16] In fact, it has also been shown to be effective with nursing students and other hospital personnel.[17,18] Tragically, nearly 14% of the nursing population experience symptoms of PTSD and as many as 33% of emergency department nurses have screened positive for PTSD.[19,20] These symptoms increase the likelihood of medical errors, which can precipitate a vicious cycle of self-doubt, fear, and blame.[21] Consequently, a female nurse is four times more likely to commit suicide than other women.[22,23] Suicide is problematic among the caregiver community, from physicians to first responders.[24,25,26] The anguish is in those who have dedicated their lives to caring are not receiving the care they have earned. For this reason alone, resilience skills are needed across the spectrum in the health care community.

One could certainly argue that this book would be helpful to anyone and the case studies could be tailored to any given group. Students today are entering college with consistently high levels of stress.[27,28] Worries about cost; employment after graduation; personal, peer, and parental pressures; and the normal developmental transition from adolescence to young adulthood make for a nerve-wracking time. And stress has been conclusively shown to have negative effects on both academic outcomes and quality of life.[29] The skills in this book address those factors or characteristics that have been repeatedly shown to improve learning while reducing the effects of negative stressors: belief in one's ability to complete tasks and reach a goal (self-efficacy), control, planning, low anxiety, and persistence.[30]

The World Health Organization focuses on resilience at individual and community levels by recognizing the role of protective factors. Repeatedly, reliably, the most important protective factor is the development and maintenance of a healthy support system.[31]

The role of spirituality can also play an important role in increasing our resilience. Spiritual practices provide us access to a socially cohesive and supportive community with a shared set of values, and lifestyle practices of positive coping strategies, good self-esteem, self-efficacy, and effective problem-solving skills. Such settings provide us opportunities to reach out and find help when needed.[32,33] And, as an aside, having a mind-set rather than a rigid one can be a protective factor as well.[34,35,36]

There is one last *why* that I need to mention. Having worked in the world of psychological trauma, I have worked with men, women, and children who have survived or been witness to horrific events. Sadly, some of us become victims of these incidents and are forever defined by what happened. But some of us become survivors of those experiences and learn to grow from them.[37,38] Do we, in fact, have the capability to thrive?

Our answer is *yes*!

The events can never be changed; what happened, happened. However, with the right skills we can navigate to a place of resilience and post-traumatic growth rather than be impaired by the tragedies that will inevitably confront us.[39,40] To be a *survivor* demands an internal commitment to learn the life lessons hidden within the heartbreaks we will encounter in our lives. To be a *survivor* requires that we practice the skills that help us maintain a healthy support system. As humans we are herd animals, and by joining together we have been able to survive as a species. The "lone wolf" is a Hollywood myth. A healthy support system is one in which we both give and receive support.

However, at this point the most important question is "*Why* are *you* reading this book?" What is motivating you? What are the internal motivators that are driving you? What are those passions that move you to action? What are the external motivators that push you? Keep your *why* in mind as you go through this book and as you practice the skills to become more resilient.

In fact, I would ask you to write down your answer. Research has shown that by writing, not by using an iPad or other devices, we activate more of our brain, recall more efficiently, and encode learning more deeply.[40,41,42]

Why am I reading this book?

_____

_____

_____

HOW

Despite our supposed sophistication, the reality is there is still a stigma associated with mental health, or if you would prefer, behavioral health. And this is even more so in the first responder community and caring professions, not to mention the military.[43,44,45,46] This book is the next iteration of a course that was designed specifically to avoid pathologizing our responses to stress and instead focus on educational practices that provide opportunities for awareness and learning without stigma. Think of this as a program about mental armor and cognitive agility and about educating ourselves to become more resilient. It is a way to understand and practice resilience skills to manage stress in a way that supports us in the development of individual and professional excellence. Those who practice resilience skills are better able to cope with the stressors that confront them.[47,48]

But please go into this knowing that succeeding will require a commitment to honestly explore attitudes and behaviors that promote or hinder the ability to grow and learn. We will ask you to challenge long-held beliefs about how one views oneself, other people, and the world. For those in the caregiving community, I would remind you of this quote:

> *The expectation that we can be immersed in suffering*
> *and loss daily, and not be touched by it, is as unrealistic as*
> *expecting to able to walk through water without getting wet.*
>
> — Rachel Naomi Remen, MD

While this quote may only apply to the medical and public service community, I am reminded of a more universal quote for students and, in fact, all of us:

> *The gem cannot be polished without friction,*
> *nor man be perfected without trials.*
>
> — Danish proverb

Life and the events we encounter, both personally and professionally, will change us. More often than not, we will not have any control over the situations; but we do have control over what we make of those events and their impact on us. Being resilient does not mean we are Pollyannaish or have a "don't worry, be happy" attitude. It means we need to recognize our internal and external resources and utilize them to deal with life's setbacks, failures, losses, and mistakes.

There is a substantial body of evidence-based research supporting both resilience and effective learning practices. The skills presented here are representative of this research along with an earnest attempt to recognize and cite some of the representative authors and studies.

Because social support is foundational to resilience, the learning of these materials in a setting where social interaction can occur and can be developed into a social support system is encouraged. In other words, try to dive in here with others, as a group. The skills are organized and delivered in a manner that is consistent with research supporting academic resilience. The process is optimized for learning while minimizing stressful distractors. Working with such a group will help keep the focus on the skills. And comparing perspectives will indeed help.

CURRICULUM

When we began to develop this curriculum we wanted to create a course where the instructional design encouraged personal interaction and had a learner-centered education format that fostered both social and scholastic resilience.[49] The notion of reflection and problem solving will be further encouraged through the use of a technique known as think-aloud pair problem solving (TAPPS).[50,51,52] When performing TAPPS, one individual verbally presents an idea while the other listens and offers feedback about the clarity and thoroughness of the idea. TAPPS aids in the development of empathy through analytical reasoning and encourages social interaction by allowing for the mutual exploration of an idea to produce deeper understanding. While designed for pairs, groups of three or even four can also be effective, especially when the individuals plan to stay together as a long-term study-support group.

We have all had courses where the material never seems relevant to our other courses. Who hasn't gone to a math class and then attended a class in something like chemistry, music, painting, or sculpture, and felt that the two courses had no connection to each other? Actually we are now uncovering just how interconnected they really are.[53,54] So when we developed the SERV course classes, we used the concepts of whole-task objectives and themes in different contexts to strengthen the idea of transfer of learning in a practical way.[55]

As this resilience curriculum has evolved to meet the special circumstances of first responders, we found that encapsulating each skill into a module facilitated the unique situation each firehouse, EMS, or police department encounters. For example, a rural volunteer department may only review a skill at a monthly training meeting, while a training academy can disseminate it on a daily basis, or a university can offer it as a credit-bearing course. Each module can be introduced and explored in just under an hour and is presented in the following manner:

1. *Review prior skills* (0–5 minutes). You and others in your group will identify any previously discussed skills and provide a very brief definition of any such skills. The process of verbalizing key points of the prior skills improves our retention, identifies functionally useful information, and situates a skill within the overall context of the skill set.[56,57]

2. *Introduce the skill* (10–15 minutes). The introduction is the content component of the skill and presented as *why* the skill is important to resilience. The skill is then processed as a procedure, recipe, guideline, or algorithm describing how the skill can be implemented. A case study will be used to situate the skill and provide an example of how the case is translated into the skill algorithm. This method promotes relevant learning through experience or experiential learning.[58] The 10–15 minutes is intended to limit lecture time and avoid the "sage on the stage." The overall point is to facilitate interaction among the group.

3. *Recollect a prior use of the skill* (5–10 minutes). Recalling recognizes that when knowledge is too tightly bound to context, transfer to different situations is reduced.[59,60,61] Therefore, to make the skills more useful, they will be explored in multiple contexts. This includes recalling a past personal experience where the skill, or something close to it, was used with some degree of success. This is the most basic of experiential learning. This internalizing is intended to build upon prior learning and any such successes, which increases our belief in ourselves or self-efficacy.[62]

There is a fun exercise we can use to illustrate why prior learning is important in new learning. First, have the people in your group say their names out loud in unison. Ask again, but encourage a louder effort. Next, hold up a piece of white paper and ask the group what color the paper is. As soon as they answer, quickly follow this with the question, "What do cows drink?" Most of us will answer "milk" rather than "water." This is referred to as associative learning.[63] Knowing that we have used a particular skill before is empowering.

Following this recalling exercise, the skill will be applied to another person through a group problem-solving exercise. We believe that learning must be relevant to our lives and must have application not just for ourselves but also for others. Next, the skill will be applied to a current personal situation.

Finally, we will apply it to a community of individuals. Focusing on a past success using the skill, current applications, as well as the vicarious experience of seeing others' experiences using the skill, will enhance the possibilities of improving upon our self-efficacy.[64,65]

Writing notes about the skill is encouraged. Expressive writing, even when written in third person, has demonstrated psychological and physical health benefits.[66,67,68]

4. *Apply the skill as a group* (5–10 minutes). This part of the presentation is intended to explore the application of the skill with another person using group problem-based learning. Up to this point, you could have examined this resilience skill on your own, but you are now asked to work with one or more people. This act of externalizing recognizes the value of different perspectives. Problem-based learning, as a group exercise, also appreciates the role of the individual and the support that is provided by others in the group.[69] Each problem that you will grapple with will be presented as a case study. As you work though this section, consider developing your own case studies that are relevant to your life and work.

I have drawn on case studies that are used in a nursing program and an EMS department that is in the area known as Hurricane Alley, to illustrate how you can create case studies that will be germane to you and your group. I have also used some different case studies in the accompanying workbook to show that you can develop scenarios that are unique to your situation.

Life is malleable. Even the most basic organism responds to the environment such that an activating event yields a consequence. If the consequence is good, the organism survives. Consequence emerges from decision. Sandwiched between the activating event and consequence is a pivotal belief—the decision mechanism. Beliefs can range from healthy to entirely self-defeating. That we are able to recognize a belief means we can control it. If we control the belief, then we control the consequence, too. We cannot control the activating event. When it happens, it happens. But we can control how we respond to it. To modify a belief is to change a consequence, to redefine self, and to adapt.

Only when we recognize the consequences of our beliefs do they have personal meaning. Identifying healthy, and especially self-defeating, beliefs is a process of observing each consequence and activating event.

Identifying the belief, when observed in another individual, requires an empathic extension beyond oneself to another individual. To do this, we must suspend our own beliefs and begin to interpret those of another person. We must walk the walk of another. Empathy is not sympathy. Rather, empathy is a survival skill that allows us critical insight into another's world. This insight can then support our efforts to create a bridge to understanding.

To communicate effectively is to coordinate an interaction with the expectation of mutual understanding or recognition of each other's beliefs. By empathizing, we work to find common ground for our beliefs, establishing a bridge to communicate and to reach out to another person. Empathy also allows someone to reach out to us. The opportunity is one of mutual respect, perhaps even support (fig. I–1).

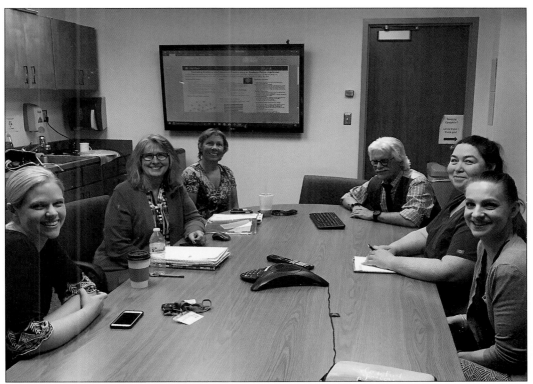

Fig. I–1. We need each other to solve life issues and cannot do it alone. (Courtesy of W. Michael Marks)

Consequently, we will work together to learn how to function in a group attempting to solve relevant life issues.

5. *Review the skill* (5 minutes). The review is intended to encourage multiple group discussions regarding the results of any prior exercises in order to address any needed clarifications, all while promoting self-efficacy. The review is to provide us an opportunity to reflect upon the process of personal and group development. Our work will not be complete until we recognize the importance of mindful and credible communication and feedback to diminish stressful situations.

6. *Practice the skill* (5–10 minutes). This time focuses on recognizing that we need to practice the skill. William Osler, who is regarded as the father of modern American medicine, observed, "Learn to see, learn to hear, learn to feel, learn to smell, and know that by practice alone you can become expert." Whereas recollecting a past application of any skill is intended to look backwards, this exercise explores our skill in the context of a current personal situation. If desired, we can explore this skill in a problem-based learning setting benefiting from the support and insight provided by others in the group.

7. *Apply the skill to a community* (5–10 minutes). The intent of this exercise is to begin to think about how to apply the skill to others in our support system and our community. Each of us needs to define community for ourselves. For example, some of us may consider our family a community, or our peer group, or work colleagues. Again, support is to be provided for and by others in the group, and our accountability to them ensures success in completing the skill. This exercise is intended to stimulate

further thought on the usefulness of the skill to others. It is also intended to reinforce the concept that a healthy support system or community is one from which we both receive and offer support.

8. *Remembering the skill* (5 minutes). Remembering is intended to provide a review of the skill and to associate some key words or phrases that help succinctly define the skill and make it easier to remember. For example, the acronym SMART (Specific, Measurable, Attainable, Realistic, Timely) is an easy reminder for the task of goal setting. Additionally, thoughtful application will be placed on mentoring and describing the skill to others to build our sense of self-efficacy.

These skills are best learned in an atmosphere that encourages social interaction. Because social support is arguably one of the most effective protections from the debilitating effects of stress, social interaction through skill learning is arguably the most appropriate method to facilitate this process. We become an active part of a social support system that grapples, through controlled exercises, with typical stressful situations that might arise in life. Does this mean that learning done in isolation is ineffective? No, certainly any effort to bring about awareness and learning is desirable. But recognize that the skills are intended to both impact the individual and sustain the individual's social support system.

Beyond our own needs are those of the community, particularly so in post-disaster psychosocial intervention. Although there are gaps in evidence-based practice, the literature currently emphasizes stress-resistant and resilience outcomes relative to promoting a sense of safety, calmness, a sense of self and community, self-efficacy, social connectedness, and hope.[70] Through your own practice of resilience, you will have an opportunity to be ready to mentor not only each other, but also your families and communities.

WHAT

The original text had a dozen skills that focused on behavior, cognition, and the development of a healthy social support system. Through continued research and development, this program has been refined to eight skills.

Throughout this program, we use a Subjective Unit of Distress Scale (SUDS) to self-evaluate the impact of a certain skill on your stress level. We encourage you to use the following scale, which is based on the one developed by South African psychiatrist Joseph Wolpe in 1969:

10 = Feeling unbearably bad, beside yourself, out of control as in a nervous breakdown, overwhelmed, at the end of your rope. You may feel so upset that you can't even talk.

9 = Feeling desperate. What most people call a 10 is actually a 9. Feeling extremely freaked out to the point that it almost feels unbearable and you are scared of what you might do. You don't want to talk because you can't imagine how anyone could possibly understand your agitation. Feeling very, very bad or losing control of your emotions.

8 = Freaking out. The beginning of alienation.

7 = Starting to freak out, on the edge of some definitely bad feelings. You can maintain control with difficulty.

6 = Feeling bad to the point that you begin to think something ought to be done about the way you feel.

5 = Moderately upset, uncomfortable. Unpleasant feelings are still manageable with some effort.

4 = Somewhat upset to the point that you cannot easily ignore an unpleasant thought. You can handle it okay but don't feel good.

3 = Mildly upset. Worried, bothered to the point that you notice it.

2 = A little bit upset, but not noticeable unless you took care to pay attention to your feelings and then realize, "yes, there is something bothering me."

1 = No acute distress and feeling basically good. If you took special effort you might feel something unpleasant, but not much.

0 = Peace, serenity, total relief. No anxiety of any kind about any particular issue.

Remember that each of us is different and someone's 4 might be another's 7. The important thing to keep in mind is that it is a means of identifying and communicating your perceptions. It is also a tool for marking progress.

RESILIENCE SKILLS

Our resilience skills begin with simple behaviors and transition to more complex cognitive and social constructs (fig. I–2). The resilience skills are identified as follows:

- *Goal setting.* Purposefully setting a goal and organizing the steps to achieve that goal provides the opportunities to mark progress, make adjustments, and build self-efficacy.

- *Fitness.* Fitness is a state of well-being and health that results from attention to and application of proper nutrition, exercise, and rest.

- *Relaxation.* Relaxation is a state of being or an act that reduces tension and stress through processes that lower metabolic rate. Maybe you already practice relaxation as an aid for getting to sleep.

- *Perspective.* One of the more powerful ways to reduce stress is to change the way you perceive an event.

- *Belief building.* Thoughts and beliefs are modifiable. Identifying and modifying self-defeating thoughts or beliefs that might bring about undesirable consequences can lower stress.

- *Thriving.* Reflecting upon the meanings of our perceived wins and fails encourages resilience by recognizing the importance of crucible events in our lives.

- *Empathy.* Empathy allows one to understand and anticipate the perceptions and perspectives of another being, making it possible to anticipate their probable future actions. Empathy provides a tried-and-true opportunity to reach out and foster communication.

- *Social support.* Social support is considered one of the best protections from suicide, PTSD, and the effects of stress.

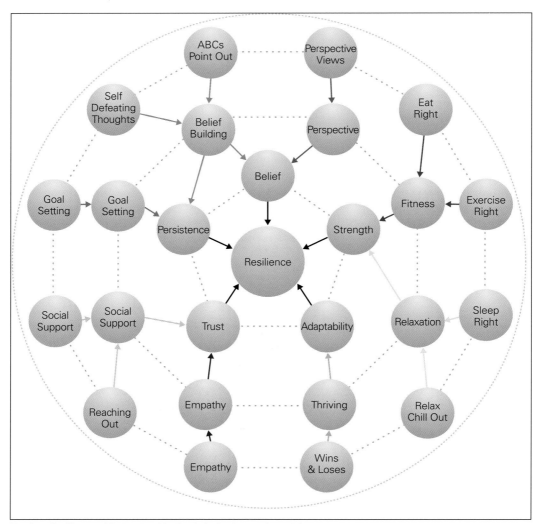

Fig. I–2. Resilience skills begin with simple behaviors and transition to more complex cognitive and social constructs.

FINAL NOTE

A hero is somebody who voluntarily walks into the unknown.

—Tom Hanks

We are all heroes in our own stories and this is even more so for those of us who are called to be of service (fig. I–3). Joseph Campbell, the American scholar and comparative mythologist, titled his most influential work *The Hero with a Thousand Faces* for good reason. You have the face of a hero, as do I. The parent who rises in the middle of the night to care for a sick child has the face of a hero. The teacher who inspires students to achieve their dreams is a hero. The first responder who runs toward the danger while others are seeking safety has the face of a hero. The nurse who holds the hand of a dying patient has the face of a hero. The child who intervenes when another kid is being bullied is a hero. Heroes come in all shapes and sizes, and more often than not, heroes don't like being called heroes.

As heroes, each of us must undertake our own personal hero's journey. This course will be such an adventure. Let us begin, together.

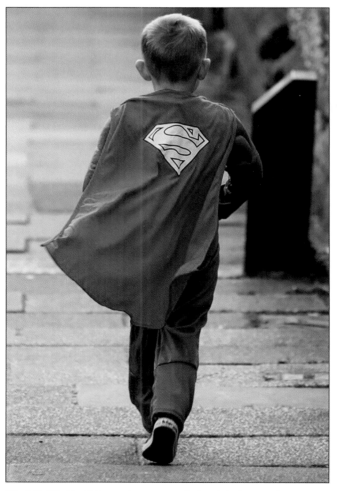

Fig. I–3. We are all heroes in our own stories. (pixabay.com)

NOTES

1   Callahan, Philip and Michael Marks. *Scholars in Camo*. Tucson: University of Arizona Press, 2008.

2   Lifton, Donald, Sandra Seay, Nancy McCarly, Rebecca Olive-Taylor, Richard Seeger, and Dalton Bigbee. "Correlating hardiness with graduation persistence." *Academic Exchange Quarterly* 10, no. 3 (2006): 277-283.

3   Sheard, Michael and Jim Golby. "Hardiness and undergraduate academic study: The moderating role of commitment." *Personality and Individual Differences* 43, no. 3 (2007): 579-588.

4   Wilks, Scott E. "Resilience amid academic stress: The moderating impact of social support among social work students." *Advances in Social Work* 9, no. 2 (2008): 106-125.

5   Markel, Nicholas, Ralph Trujillo, Philip Callahan, and Michael Marks. "Resiliency and retention in veterans returning to college: Results of a pilot study" [presentation]. Veterans in Higher Education Conference: Listening, Responding and Changing for Student Success. Sept. 2010. Tucson, AZ.

6   Benedek, David M., Carol Fullerton, and Robert J. Ursano. "First responders: Mental health consequences of natural and human-made disasters for public health and public safety workers." *Annual Review of Public Health* 28 (2007): 55-68.

7   Fullerton, Carol S., Robert J. Ursano, and Leming Wang. "Acute stress disorder, posttraumatic stress disorder, and depression in disaster or rescue workers." *American Journal of Psychiatry* 161, no. 8 (2004): 1370-1376.

8   Foa, Edna B., Terence M. Keane, Matthew J. Friedman, and Judith A. Cohen, eds. *Effective Treatments for PTSD: Practice Guidelines from the International Society for Traumatic Stress Studies*. New York: Guilford Press, 2008.

9   Kang, Han K., Tim A. Bullman, Derek J. Smolenski, Nancy A. Skopp, Gregory A. Gahm, and Mark A. Reger. "Suicide risk among 1.3 million veterans who were on active duty during the Iraq and Afghanistan wars." *Annals of Epidemiology* 25, no. 2 (2015): 96-100.

10 Stanley, Ian H., Melanie A. Hom, and Thomas E. Joiner. "A systematic review of suicidal thoughts and behaviors among police officers, firefighters, EMTs, and paramedics." *Clinical Psychology Review* 44, no. 3 (2016): 25-44.

11 Newland, Chad, Erich Barber, Monique Rose, and Amy Young. "Survey reveals alarming rates of EMS provider stress and thoughts of suicide." *Journal of Emergency Medical Services* 40, no. 10 (2015): 30-34.

12 Tiesman, Hope M., Srinivas Konda, Dan Hartley, Cammie Chaumont Menéndez, Marilyn Ridenour, and Scott Hendricks. "Suicide in US workplaces, 2003–2010: A comparison with non-workplace suicides." *American Journal of Preventive Medicine* 48, no. 6 (2015): 674-682.

13 World Health Organization. *Preventing Suicide: A Resource for Police, Firefighters and Other First Line Responders*. Geneva: WHO, 2009.

14 Gunderson, Jonathan, Mike Grill, Philip Callahan, and Michael Marks. "An evidence-based program for improving and sustaining first responder behavioral health." *Journal of Emergency Medical Services* 39, no. 3 (2014): 57-61.

15 Lo Giudice, Tony A. and Jeff Dyar. "MEMS Resilience Training." Metropolitan Emergency Medical Services [Little Rock, AR], www.metroems.org, Oct. 2016.

16 Marks, Michael. "Colorado Office of Emergency Preparedness and Response: Resilience Report." Colorado Department of Public Health and Environment, www.colorado.gov, Dec. 2016.

17 Wilger, P., Kosanke, H., Bouchard, L., Pasquet, C., Williams, D., Oja, K., Callahan, P., Marks, M.W., and Larson, W. "Developing Professional Resiliency in Pre-Licensure Nursing Students" [abstract]. Arizona Nurses Association Symposium: Healthy Nurse, Healthy Patient, Healthy Nation. Phoenix, AZ, Oct. 2016.

18 Lo Giudice, Tony A. "Hospital based resilience: A pathway to combating stress." *Arizona Hospital and Healthcare Association*, Marana, AZ, June 2016.

19 Mealer, Meredith, Ellen L. Burnham, Colleen J. Goode, Barbara Rothbaum, and Marc Moss. "The prevalence and impact of post traumatic stress disorder and burnout syndrome in nurses." *Depression and Anxiety* 26, no. 12 (2009): 1118-1126.

20 Kerasiotis, Bernadina and Robert W. Motta. "Assessment of PTSD symptoms in emergency room, intensive care unit, and general floor nurses." *International Journal of Emergency Mental Health* 6, no. 3 (2003): 121-133.

21 Rassin, Michal, Tammy Kanti, and Dina Silner. "Chronology of medication errors by nurses: Accumulation of stresses and PTSD symptoms." *Issues in Mental Health Nursing* 26, no. 8 (2005): 873-886.

22 Alderson, Marie, Xavier Parent-Rocheleau, and Brian Mishara. "Critical review on suicide among nurses: What about work-related factors?" *Crisis: The Journal of Crisis Intervention and Suicide Prevention* 36, no. 2 (2015): 91-101.

23 American Society of Registered Nurses. "Nurses at risk." *Nursing Today,* http://www.asrn.org/journal-nursing-today/291-nurses-at-risk.html, Feb. 2008.

24 Center, Claudia, Miriam Davis, Thomas Detre, Daniel E. Ford, Wendy Hansbrough, Herbert Hendin, John Laszlo et al. "Confronting Depression and suicide in physicians: A consensus statement." *Journal of American Medical Association* 289, no. 23 (2003): 3161-3166.

25 Stanley, Ian H., Melanie A. Hom, and Thomas E. Joiner. "A systematic review of suicidal thoughts and behaviors among police officers, firefighters, EMTs, and paramedics." *Clinical Psychology Review* 44, no. 3 (2016): 25-44.

26 Newland, Chad, Erich Barber, Monique Rose, and Amy Young. "Survey reveals alarming rates of EMS provider stress and thoughts of suicide." *Journal of Emergency Medical Services* 40, no. 10 (2015): 30-34.

27 Pryor, John H., Sylvia Hurtado, Linda DeAngelo, Laura Palucki Blake, and Serge Tran. *The American Freshman: National Norms Fall 2010.* Los Angeles: Higher Education Research Institute, UCLA, 2010.

28 Pryor, John H., Kevin Eagan, Laura Palucki Blake, Sylvia Hurtado, Jennifer Berdan, and Mathew H. Case. *The American Freshman: National Norms Fall 2012.* Los Angeles: Higher Education Research Institute, UCLA, 2012.

29 DeBerard, M. Scott, Glen I. Spielmans, and Deana L. Julka. "Predictors of academic achievement and retention among college freshmen: A longitudinal study." *College Student Journal* 38, no. 1 (2004): 66.

30 Martin, Andrew J. and Herbert W. Marsh. "Academic resilience and its psychological and educational correlates: A construct validity approach." *Psychology in the Schools* 43, no. 3 (2006): 267-281.

31 Brewin, Chris R., Bernice Andrews, and John D. Valentine. "Meta-analysis of risk factors for posttraumatic stress disorder in trauma-exposed adults." *Journal of Consulting and Clinical Psychology* 68, no. 5 (2000): 748.

32 Peres, Julio F.P., Alexander Moreira-Almeida, Antonia Gladys Nasello, and Harold G. Koenig. "Spirituality and resilience in trauma victims." *Journal of Religion and Health* 46, no. 3 (2007): 343-350.

33 Benson, Jill and Jill Thistlethwaite. *Mental Health Across Cultures: A Practical Guide for Health Professionals.* Boca Raton, FL: CRC Press, 2009.

34 Tugade, Michele M., Barbara L. Fredrickson, and Lisa Feldman Barrett. "Psychological resilience and positive emotional granularity: Examining the benefits of positive emotions on coping and health." *Journal of Personality* 72, no. 6 (2004): 1161-1190.

35 Abe, Jo Ann A. "Positive emotions, emotional intelligence, and successful experiential learning." *Personality and Individual Differences* 51, no. 7 (2011): 817-822.

36 Fresco, Nancy and Kristin Timm. "Fostering resilience in the face of an uncertain future: Using scenario planning to communicate climate change risks and collaboratively develop adaptation strategies." In *Communicating Climate-Change and Natural Hazard Risk and Cultivating Resilience.* Cham: Springer International Publishing, 2016, 79-94.

37 Calhoun, Lawrence G. and Richard G. Tedeschi. *Handbook of Posttraumatic Growth: Research and Practice.* New York: Routledge/Tayor & Francis, 2014.

38 Schiraldi, Glenn R. *The Post-Traumatic Stress Disorder Sourcebook: A Guide to Healing, Recovery, and Growth.* New York: McGraw Hill Professional, 2009.

39 Bloom, Sandra L. "By the crowd they have been broken, by the crowd they shall be healed: The social transformation of trauma." In *Posttraumatic Growth: Positive Changes in the Aftermath of Crisis.* Mahwah, NJ: Erlbaum, 1998, 179-213.

40 Klein, Kitty and Adriel Boals. "Expressive writing can increase working memory capacity." *Journal of Experimental Psychology: General* 130, no. 3 (2001): 520-533.

41 Andersson, Mathew A. and Coleen S. Conley. "Optimizing the perceived benefits and health outcomes of writing about traumatic life events." *Stress and Health* 29, no. 1 (2013): 40-49.

42 Torrance, Mark and David Galbraith. "The processing demands of writing." In *Handbook of Writing Research.* New York: Guilford Press, 2006, 67-80.

43 Wahl, Otto and Eli Aroesty-Cohen. "Attitudes of mental health professionals about mental illness: A review of the recent literature." *Journal of Community Psychology* 38, no. 1 (2010): 49-62.

44 Sheppard, Kate. "Compassion fatigue among registered nurses: Connecting theory and research." *Applied Nursing Research* 28, no. 1 (2015): 57-59.

45 Clement, Sarah, Oliver Schauman, Tanya Graham, F. Maggioni, Sara Evans-Lacko, Nikita Bezborodovs, Craig Morgan, Nicolas Rüsch, June S. L. Brown, and Graham Thornicroft. "What is the impact of mental health-related stigma on help-seeking? A systematic review of quantitative and qualitative studies." *Psychological Medicine* 45, no. 1 (2015): 11-27.

46 Henderson, Sarah N., Vincent B. Van Hasselt, Todd J. LeDuc, and Judy Couwels. "Firefighter suicide: Understanding cultural challenges for mental health professionals." *Professional Psychology: Research and Practice* 47, no. 3 (2016): 224-230.

47   Edward, Karen-leigh and Philip Warelow. "Resilience: When coping is emotionally intelligent." *Journal of the American Psychiatric Nurses Association* 11, no. 2 (2005): 101-102.

48   Mayordomo, Teresa, Paz Viguer, Alicia Sales, Encarnación Satorres, and Juan C. Meléndez. "Resilience and coping as predictors of well-being in adults." *The Journal of Psychology* 150, no. 7 (2016): 809-821.

49   Weimer, Maryellen. *Learner Centered Teaching: Five Key Changes to Practice*. San Francisco: John Wiley and Sons, 2013.

50   Barkley, Elizabeth F., K. Patricia Cross, and Claire Howell Major. *Collaborative Learning Techniques: A Handbook for College Faculty*. San Francisco: Jossey-Bass, 2005.

GOAL SETTING

A dream without a goal is just a wish.

— Antoine de Saint-Exupéry

OVERVIEW

Why: Goal setting is the process of developing an organized plan to achieve a defined and attainable result. Purposefully setting a goal and taking the steps to achieve that goal is a way we can mark progress, make adjustments, and build *self-efficacy*—the belief in one's abilities.

How: When we write a goal and the series of steps needed to satisfy the goal, it needs to be such that when all of the steps are completed the goal has been attained.

Use the following guidelines for goal setting:

- The goal statement must be directed to only the task at hand.
  - It should be Specific, Measurable, Attainable, Realistic, and Timely (SMART).
- Write it in such a manner that you will see your goal's completion.
- The steps are to identify the key actions that are necessary to attain the goal.
  - It is intended to assure an adequate number of steps are included to mark your progress.
  - Don't overlook the fact that each step is to be written so that your completion of each step is obvious.
- The steps can then be checked off (✓) as each is completed and a reward should be available (and savored).

Usually when we first think about achieving a goal there is a certain amount of nervousness and anticipation about being able to accomplish it. We may get excited about the possibilities, but not really consider the obstacles we may confront. Or we may start thinking about all of the reasons we won't be able to attain the goal.[1,2,3] Think of a goal you'd like to reach and reflect on what happens.

Identifying a measure of change between before and after developing the goal and the steps to meet the goal provides us with a way to measure our success. Here, we suggest the use of the Subjective Units of Distress Scale (SUDS) to help you subjectively identify your stress levels before setting a goal and again after the goal is attained. The levels are somewhere between zero (0) and ten (10), where 0 corresponds to no stress and 10 to the highest level of stress you have ever experienced. The anticipation is that the SUDS level begins to decrease even after developing a goal statement and the steps to attain the goal. If your SUDS level increases, then take some time to reassess your goal statement to assure it is attainable. And reassess the steps to assure that they have been adequately defined and there are as many as you need. After all, you want to be able to check off each step and mark progress toward reaching your goal.

Goal-Setting Skill

The whole idea here is to help you address your stress. That starts by recognizing your present perceived stress level. Some people think verbally, some think visually (like me), and some think mathematically. Use the style that best suits you.

Rate the stress level you perceive

Analog SUDS	Digital SUDS	Emoji SUDS
Actually, I'm not stressed	0	😃
A little stressed	1–3	🙂
Somewhat stressed	4–6	😐
Quite a bit stressed	7–8	😟
It's really bad	9	🙁
Run and hide!	10	😫

Think about what's stressing you out. What might help?

Try and identify an objective to help you do that.

Now it's time to figure out how to get there.

Write out your goal statement and how you plan to get there, step-by-step.

Now get started! Don't be shy. Go for it!

Have you made any progress?

Rate the stress level you perceive now

Is it lower?

Yes	No
👍 Congratulations, you did it! Now you can do this whenever you need it!	What might have gone wrong? Did you figure out all your steps? Did you actually do them all? Did you give yourself enough time? Give it another try, from the beginning.

Is SUDS the only option for measuring change? Certainly not! You are encouraged to find the most appropriate measurement for your needs. The only thing that matters is that it can provide meaningful feedback with regard to change, or even transformation, resulting from applying the goal-setting process. Perhaps a scale that measures the likelihood of completing the task might be more useful. That scale might range from 0 to 10, where 0 corresponds to zero chance of completion and 10 is fully sure of completion. If you were using a likelihood-of-completion scale, then you would anticipate an increase in likelihood to complete from premeasure to postmeasure.

WHY GOAL SETTING?

What keeps me going is goals.

— Muhammad Ali

We all set goals every day. Even getting out of bed in the morning can be a goal. The first step usually begins with turning off the alarm. This is followed by some inspirational and motivating self-talk like, "Get your sorry ass outta bed."

When we reach our goals, it is essential that we take time to reward and acknowledge our successes. Even if it is just sitting with our first cup of coffee and praising ourselves for not hitting the snooze button one more time.

It is important for us to understand how we set goals and what motivates us to achieve them. For some of us, there are internal drives that inspire us to achieve our goals. For others, it may be external forces that push us. For most of us it is a combination. What motivates you to achieve your goals?

Goals and goal setting have a history of research spanning decades and disciplines that include leadership, education, and psychology. The notion of goal setting emerged as a recognition of the role of conscious intent as a motivational cause.[4,5,6]

Wouldn't it be great if we would spend as much time planning our lives as we do planning a vacation? What would your life look like if you planned it as meticulously as you do a vacation?

One of the greatest values of setting and achieving goals is the impact on our self-discipline and self-esteem.[7,8] Self-discipline and self-esteem go hand in hand. Once we understand how self-discipline (making our bed every morning) increases our self-esteem (I accomplished a goal I've set for myself), we grow to appreciate how important self-discipline is in our lives.[9,10]

Research in human motivation has determined that of all the motivational drivers in the workplace (including accomplishment/completion, earned recognition, career advancement, and even personal self-development), accomplishment nearly always comes out on top.[11,12,13]

Even on a neurobiological level, reaching a goal or even completing a step to a goal can have remarkable reinforcing consequences for us. In fact, some suggest that our brains actually desire completion, because by doing so we set up the release of a chain of pleasure chemicals. And by not completing a task, we can trigger a flood of stress chemicals into our brains.[14,15]

Given its early history in industrial-organizational psychology, *goal setting* might be broadly defined as the conscious development of a plan to guide a person or group toward a goal or desired end-point, often within some time span. Goal-setting theory considers the impact of *motivation*, the desire and intent to reach a goal. This theory argues that setting a goal implies discontent with our present condition. And, as long as our goal is attainable, there are no conflicting goals, and there is a commitment to the goal, then there is a relationship between goal difficulty and goal performance. This relationship between goal difficulty and goal performance suggests that harder goals are more motivating to us than easier goals because they require us to accomplish more in order to be satisfied.[16,17]

There are also *mediators*, which are the mechanisms through which goal setting affects performance. Specifically, goals are motivators. They impact persistence, focus attention, and activate old as well as new knowledge and even strategies.[18]

Other elements, labeled *moderators*, impact goal setting. One example of a moderator is receiving adequate feedback from others to help us to track progress and clarify the steps we need to include to reach our goal. Another moderator is our ability to establish our goal commitment, which is enhanced by self-efficacy, and to assign a goal importance. We also need to recognize that task complexity is limited by task knowledge. That is, task knowledge is more difficult to acquire as the tasks become more complex. A moderator is also our understanding of situational constraints that limit us, such as dealing with excess work without having sufficient resources.[19]

When goals are self-established, people who demonstrate higher self-efficacy set more demanding goals than those with lower self-efficacy. Further, the more self-efficacious individuals demonstrate a greater goal commitment and find better strategies to attain the goals. In particular, this is seen in the context of learning goals.[20] As learners, we are affected by our perceived goal progress, which is the path leading to goal attainment. Goal setting and self-efficacy are affected by self-observation, self-judgment, and self-reaction.[21]

The effects of self-efficacy, grade goals, and effort regulation emerge as strong predictors of course grades and grade point average (GPA).[22,23] Students who set both near- and long-term grade goals reliably show higher GPAs.[24]

Grit has appeared as a predictor of academic success. It is defined as perseverance and passion for long-term goals. Further, this is considered the effort and interest exercised toward a set goal that is positively sustained throughout the course of reaching that goal. Grit is considered a trait that can be taught and nurtured to improve self-regulation and goal success.[25,26,27]

Finally, as a psychological construct, the framing of goal setting becomes pivotal. For example, those of us who perceive the goal to be a challenge show better performance than those who perceive the goal to be threatening and potentially leading to failure.[28] Additionally, setting specific difficult goals leads us to better performance than no goals or vague goals, such as "do your best."[29] This is demonstrated in behavioral and physical health programs such as goal coaching as an approach to physical rehabilitation, dietary and exercise programs, personal development, and goal attainment.[30,31,32,33]

THE HOW OF GOAL SETTING

When it is obvious that the goals cannot be reached,
don't adjust the goals, adjust the action steps.

— Confucius

Goals can range from small to big, depending upon our perception of the goal and the resources we need to meet the goal. Making the effort to smile at people can be a goal, as can showing people that we care about them. Again, while we may set dozens of goals every day, we may not be fully aware of the implications of the act or the process we go through to attain the goal (fig. 1–1). Being able to create an attainable goal and the steps to achieve that goal has been found to increase our sense of self-efficacy, thus producing a positive loop leading to an even greater likelihood of success.[34,35,36,37]

Goal implications can have unexpected consequences. For example, unrealistic and difficult goals can lead to depression and a self-fulfilling prophecy of failure.[38] On the other hand, goals that are too easily attainable can lead to boredom and apathy about reaching the goal. Attainment can also be influenced by whether the goals are imposed on us or if we have some say in the development of the goals.[39,40]

It is important to differentiate between the notions of *goal commitment* and *goal acceptance*.[41] We may accept that studying for classes is a goal that we have to make to reach the larger goal of graduating from our program of studies. If, however, we are not committed to studying on a daily basis, we may fail to graduate. There are intrinsic and extrinsic motivations to achieving a goal.[42,43] That is, we may have internal (intrinsic) motivation to achieve a certain goal when there is no external (extrinsic) motivation to do so. Alternatively, there may be little intrinsic motivation but lots of external motivation to accomplish a goal. Most often our goal setting is derived from some combination of all these factors. Awareness of these factors better prepares us to develop a viable goal and the steps needed to attain that goal.[44,45]

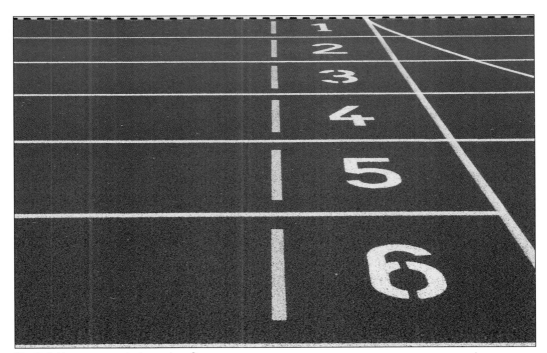

Fig. 1–1. How many goals do you have?

Time management

*You've got to know what you want. This is central to acting
on your intentions. When you know what you want,
you realize that all there is left then is time management.*

— Patch Adams, MD

Effective time management is problematic for most us and it becomes even more complicated when we have to balance family, exercise, social obligations, education, and a job (fig. 1–2). Students who perceive control of their time tend to report greater performance and life satisfaction, and less role overload and stress.[46] Time management is shown to have a greater buffering effect on academic stress than leisure activities.[47] Engaging in some time management behaviors can have beneficial effects on stress and job satisfaction.[48,49]

A goal of time management is to blend lifestyle with goal setting. A commonly used process is to identify how you are currently allocating your time and then perform an optimizing process to better address your activity and time needs. The optimizing process results in a calendar or planner that allows you to identify daily routines as well as when special events impact your daily routines. By identifying and compartmentalizing your routines and identifying important activity dates, you can establish boundaries that ultimately permit you to enjoy guilt-free personal time without the stressful thought of "I should be doing…"

Using a notebook, spreadsheet, word processor, or other recording device, create a daily calendar noting by unit of time (every 15 minutes, 30 minutes, or hour) the activity you are performing. Now, maintain this calendar for one week (table 1–1).

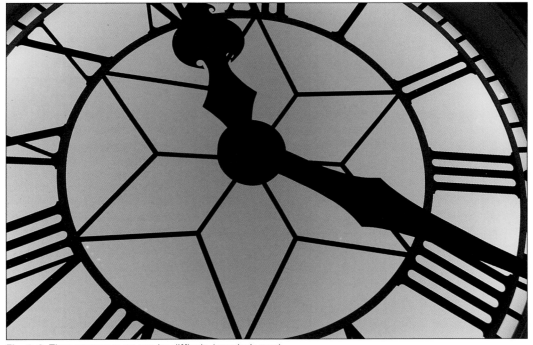

Fig. 1–2. Time management can be difficult. (unsplash.com)

> *I decide how I will complete the goal, step by step. The process is systematic. Each step brings me closer to the goal. I write each step in a manner that permits me to determine when it has been completed. The step is measured by limitation. I can check it off. I can mark progress toward goal completion. I persist.*
>
> *Marking progress builds belief, a commitment to ensure I complete the goal. I therefore write the number of steps to both mark progress and provide direction. These details ensure that I am neither lost nor mired in my journey to the goal. When I have completed all of the steps, I have attained the goal. I am ready for whatever comes next.*

What color is your ink? Put it in writing!

Table 1–1. Example of part of a calendar of personal activities

Time	Monday	Tuesday	Wednesday	Thursday
5:00	wake	wake	wake	...
15	feed pet	feed pet	feed pet	...
30	jog	walk pet	jog	...
45		water garden		...
6:00		shower		...
15	shower	breakfast	shower	...
30	breakfast	read newspaper	breakfast	...
45	bike to work	bike to work	bike to work	

At the end of that week, analyze how you used your time by identifying common activities or tasks and the time spent on these. Activities to consider should also include free time for family or social activities. But that doesn't mean you can ignore classes, work, study, meals (and their preparation), exercise, and chores. The intent of this weeklong analysis is to create an organized calendar or a planner that indicates time spent on key activities. For example, identify an adequate amount of free time while assuring that you put your most mentally demanding tasks into time slots that make the best use of your mental and physical resources. Your planner should be a tool that accommodates your lifestyle.

Summarizing:

1. The weekly time log documents the time you are actually spending on tasks and activities as you progress through the week.

2. It also situates the recurring activities appearing in your weekly time log, such that your days are presented in an optimized manner allowing repetitive activities to be identified.

3. Task goals and the steps to attain these goals are elements that may or may not immediately appear within the organized weekly calendar. They can and should be added as they arise.

   a. Consider setting goals and objectives for work projects. These can be blended into the organized weekly calendar to become a daily planner.

4. Blend the activities of task goals and objectives into the calendar to organize your time into an adaptable daily planner.

5. The next step is to actually translate this information into some sort of daily planner. Your planner should be a tool that accommodates your lifestyle. Consider using a simple form such as a small notebook, a wall calendar, a commercially printed daily planner with calendar, or a more sophisticated tool such as a software application for your cell phone and that lets you share data with others. Pick the tool that you will use.

Time management provides an opportunity to practice goal setting!

> *This is the key to time management—to see the value of every moment.*
>
> — Menachem Mendel Schneerson

A method for goal setting

A frequently used term in psychology, *successive approximation*, refers to the ongoing shaping of behavior as new information comes in, helping guide us toward a desired end.[50] The same can be said for goal setting. A *goal* is often defined as the conscious development of a plan to guide a person (or group) toward a desired result. It is important to develop a realistic objective along with the smaller and more manageable steps required to attain it. The purpose of these steps is to help eliminate any ambiguity by providing limitations to the broader intention. These steps can also introduce more flexibility in attaining the aspiration.[51]

Steps also provide a mechanism for ongoing self-evaluation.[52] They provide opportunities for rewards along the way of attaining your larger goal. Too often we focus only on the goal and miss the intrinsic and extrinsic values associated with satisfying the smaller steps toward meeting their purpose. Put another way, we forget to stop and smell the roses.

Are there other options for goal setting? While the method described here does provide a reliable how-to of the basics of goal setting, finding other tools such as dedicated apps for goal setting might be beneficial. The goal, of course, is to complete the goal setting. If you should find a more appropriate tool that moves you to completion, then use it.

Examples of goal setting

I already know I am going into a high-stress career. I am also in an applied program of studies that is considered high stress. After reading some of the stress-related research, I have decided to take a resilience class. The class I selected meets only once as an all-day classroom session. The classroom session is on *resilience skill awareness* and includes some preliminary focus on the application of the skills. The expectation, though, is that I will apply and practice these skills as identified exercises after the classroom session and submit the work for class credit.

There are a total of eight resilience skills, and each skill has four exercises: two focusing on self and two focusing on people with whom you associate.

I need to identify at least one other person who will work with me on these exercises so we can assure each of us completes them.

My program of studies is demanding. I want to complete these exercises within a month of the classroom session, and I want to use goal setting to assure I successfully complete everything on time.

Because I intend to complete the task with two other people, I will work on this using the think-aloud pair problem solving (TAPPS) approach. TAPPS is a collaborative problem-solving process where individuals work in pairs or a team. The problem victim talks through a problem or challenge, and the listener (or listeners) asks questions relative to the problem victim's thought process. Specifically, the listener reviews and provides constructive feedback on the clarity and thoroughness of the ideas and options under consideration.[53] In this manner we assist each other in developing a goal statement and the steps needed to appropriately and successfully address the issue(s).

Although we are working collaboratively, we still have some flexibility to personalize the goal-setting skill to best meet our individual needs as well as those of the group. Having high personal goals that are compatible with the group's goal should enhance the group's performance.[54] Therefore, I establish a baseline measure before beginning the process and measure again after I write my goal and the steps to attain it. The baseline measure I am using is SUDS. By writing out the process of identifying and setting my goal, I was able to clarify my thinking and establish a series of steps that brought me to a successful conclusion to the resilience class. Not only that, but I contributed to the approaches my group intends to follow. I intend to continue to use goal setting for my program of studies to aid me in better managing my time to meet class requirements while lowering my level of stress. I hope the others will, too.

Example:

Baseline SUDS (0–10)	7	√
Goal	Complete resilience program within four weeks.	√
SUDS intensity (0–10)	5	√
Step 1	Identify a study group.	√
Step 2	Determine what needs to be completed.	?
Step 3	Identify group study times.	√
Step 4	Agree on the material(s) to be covered at each meeting.	?
Step 5	Complete first week exercises.	?
Step 6	Complete second week exercises.	?
Step 7	Complete third week exercises.	?
Step 8	Complete fourth week exercises.	?
Step 9	Submit completed work for credit.	?
Step 10	(Need more space?)	?
SUDS intensity (0–10)	_____	?

INTERNALIZE GOAL SETTING

I've worked too hard and too long to let anything stand in the way of my goals. I will not let my teammates down and I will not let myself down.

— Mia Hamm

Recall, in as much detail as possible, a past personal experience where you used goal setting to successfully address a situation.

▩ What made that goal memorable?

_____
_____
_____
_____

▩ What drove you to attain the goal?

_____
_____
_____
_____

▩ How did you attain the goal?

_____
_____
_____
_____

Given that goal-setting experience, translate it to the goal setting skill. If you prefer, consider writing a brief story about your goal setting experience and build in the goal setting skill. Work on this process individually or collaboratively. Consider using a TAPPS collaborative pair or group to assist you in writing the goal statement and the steps you performed to complete the goal.

A scoring rubric is intended to communicate expectations of quality regarding a particular task. The rubric functions as an aid or checklist for task completion and provides a basis for self-evaluation, reflection, and comparable peer review. The rubric is not intended to constrain you; rather use it as a basic checklist of learning objectives for completing this resilience skill.

Checklist for Internalizing Goal Setting

Consider a past personal situation where goal setting was used with some success.

Baseline SUDS (0–10)	_____	? √
Goal	Identify the task that was accomplished.	? √
SUDS intensity (0–10)	_____	? √
Step 1	Write the goal statement.	? √
Step 2	Write the steps that attained the goal.	? √
Step 3	Identify the time frame in which the task was completed.	? √
SUDS intensity (0–10)	_____	? √

Step 4	Did writing the goal statement make the task clearer?	? √
Step 5	Did writing the goal statement make the task more manageable?	? √
Step 6	Did writing the steps needed make the task clearer?	? √
Step 7	Did writing the steps needed make the task more manageable?	? √
Step 8	Was checking off each step as it was completed helpful?	? √
SUDS intensity (0–10) _____		? √

EXTERNALIZE: APPLY GOAL SETTING AS A GROUP

One way to keep momentum going is to have constantly greater goals.

— Michael Korda

If you are a health care provider, you already know how horrible people in this profession are at self-care and that most would rather focus on helping others.

In each resilience training session I do there is the crusty first responder or nurse who complains about all of this "fluffy resilience stuff." My response and those of my colleagues is this, "We don't care about you; we care about your spouse, children, and extended family. This is about the impact you might have on them. By learning these skills, you can better understand how you can help them cope with the fallout of your work." With that shift in focus, they become the most engaged.

This externalization exercise is intended to explore the application of the skill to another person using group problem-based learning (PBL). As a group exercise, pay particular attention to the role of the individual and the support that is provided by others in the group.[68] Each problem that you will grapple with will be presented as a case study. As you work though this section, consider developing your own case studies that are relevant to your situation.

> *I have drawn on case studies that are used in a nursing program by academic advisors and by an EMS department that is in area that commonly experiences hurricanes. The intent here is to illustrate how you can create case studies that will be germane to you and your group.*

Case study: Dennis is a nontraditional student. He is 27 years old, married, with an adorable 2-year-old daughter who has him wrapped around her finger. He works part time as a certified nursing assistant (CNA) at a long-term care facility, is in the National Guard, and is a full-time nursing student at the nearby college. He recognizes that he has lots of demands and he thinks taking a resiliency course will help him cope better with these stresses. He intends to complete the resiliency training with two other friends, but would like your input about how best to successfully complete the course. Your goal is to use goal setting to devise this plan.

Note: The following rubric is not intended to be constraining, but rather used as a basic checklist of learning objectives for applying this resilience skill.

Checklist for Externalizing Goal Setting

Preparatory	Consider whether there are family personality issues to address.	? √
Baseline SUDS (0–10)	_____	? √
Goal	Identify the task to be accomplished.	? √
SUDS intensity (0–10)	_____	? √
Clarify	What is the necessary time frame?	? √
SUDS intensity (0–10)	_____	? √
Step 1	Write the goal statement.	? √
Step 2	Write the steps to attain the goal.	? √
SUDS intensity (0–10)	_____	? √
Step 3	Did writing the goal statement make the task clearer?	? √
Step 4	Did writing the goal statement make the task more manageable?	? √
Step 5	Did writing the steps needed make the task clearer?	? √
Step 6	Did writing the steps needed make the task more manageable?	? √
Step 7	Was checking off each step as it was completed helpful?	? √
SUDS intensity (0–10)	_____	? √
Step 8	What are the prospective consequences?	? √
Step 9	Did the collaborative approach help?	? √
Step 10	Is this system something you will feel competent to use again?	? √
SUDS intensity (0–10)	_____	? √

PRACTICE GOAL SETTING

Setting goals is the first step in turning the invisible into the visible.

—Tony Robbins

One of the best ways we can really integrate a skill into our lives is to make it personal. To do this, we need to see the value of it in our lives. To put it bluntly, "What's in it for me?" You have applied this new skill format to a situation that had occurred in your past, so you have an awareness of how to use this skill. You have also applied the skill as a group PBL exercise by focusing on someone who could benefit from using this skill. Now consider how you could best apply the goal-setting skill to a current event you are facing. Practicing the skill provides an opportunity to reflect on prior learning and make the skill more personally memorable.

Checklist for Practicing Goal Setting

Current circumstances:

Baseline SUDS (0–10)	_____	?	√
Goal	Identify the task to be accomplished.	?	√
SUDS intensity (0–10)	_____	?	√
Clarify	What is the necessary time frame?	?	√
SUDS intensity (0–10)	_____	?	√
Step 1	Write the goal statement.	?	√
Step 2	Write the steps to attain the goal.	?	√
SUDS intensity (0–10)	_____	?	√
Step 3	Did writing the goal statement make the task clearer?	?	√
Step 4	Did writing the goal statement make the task more manageable?	?	√
Step 5	Did writing the steps needed make the task clearer?	?	√
Step 6	Did writing the steps needed make the task more manageable?	?	√
Step 7	Was checking off each step as it was completed helpful?	?	√
SUDS intensity (0–10)	_____	?	√
Step 8	What are the prospective consequences?	?	√
Step 9	Is this system something you will feel competent to use again?	?	√
SUDS intensity (0–10)	_____	?	√

APPLY GOAL SETTING TO YOUR COMMUNITY

*The discipline you learn and character you build from setting and achieving
a goal can be more valuable than the achievement of the goal itself.*

— Bo Bennett

The intent of this exercise is to begin to think about how to apply the skill to others in our support system and our community. Each of us needs to define community for ourselves. For example, some of us may consider our family a community. Others may consider it to be a peer group or work colleagues. Again, the support is to be provided by others in the group. Our accountability to them underscores our commitment to the success in completing the skill. This exercise is intended to stimulate further thought on the usefulness of the skill to others. It is also intended to reinforce the concept that a healthy support system, or community, is one from which we both receive and offer support.

What are the implications of expanding this skill to a community of individuals? Certainly the task becomes more complex, but recognize that you have already effectively used a collaborative group for goal setting. How do you expect this event to eventually conclude?

Checklist for Applying Goal Setting to Your Community

Community circumstances:

Baseline SUDS (0–10)	_____	?	√
Goal	Identify the task to be accomplished.	?	√
SUDS intensity (0–10)	_____	?	√
Clarify	What is the necessary time frame?	?	√
SUDS intensity (0–10)	_____	?	√
Step 1	Write the goal statement.	?	√
Step 2	Write the steps to attain the goal.	?	√
SUDS intensity (0–10)	_____	?	√
Step 3	Did writing the goal statement make the task clearer?	?	√
Step 4	Did writing the goal statement make the task more manageable?	?	√
Step 5	Did writing the steps needed make the task clearer?	?	√
Step 6	Did writing the steps needed make the task more manageable?	?	√
Step 7	Was checking off each step as it was completed helpful?	?	√
SUDS intensity (0–10)	_____	?	√
Step 8	What are the prospective consequences?	?	√
Step 9	Is this system something you will feel competent to use again?	?	√
Step 10	Will goal setting be helpful?	?	√
Step 11	How do you see the community interacting?	?	√
SUDS intensity (0–10)	_____	?	√

A challenge associated with this community goal-setting exercise is to define your community and its need. Successful goal setting can a have a profound effect on a wide variety of community endeavors that might range from collaborating with immediate family members to improving schools or to conserving energy.[55,56,57]

> *If you have raised children or are in the process of raising them, you know about school projects. Even if it is last minute, it can be an opportunity to teach the concept of goal setting to this most precious community of ours. Children can learn about the steps needed to accomplish the goal of completing their school project, including improved time management.*

REMEMBERING GOAL SETTING

You have been encouraged to examine and apply this goal-setting skill format. Take the opportunity now to reflect on the skill and think of some key words or phrases that help to succinctly define the skill (fig. 1–3). When you have completed this process, compare these key words and phrases with the person or persons with whom you are working. Discuss and decide if you wish to alter any of your reflective key words or phrases. What have you learned through this process?

_____

_____

_____

_____

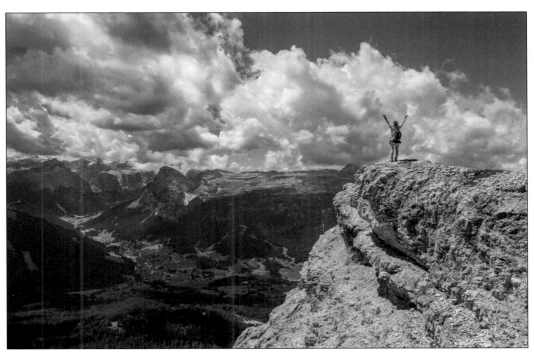

Fig. 1–3. Reaching goals leads to success. (unsplash.com)

People with goals succeed because they know where they're going.

— Earl Nightingale

NOTES

1   Eum, KoUn and Kenneth G. Rice. "Test anxiety, perfectionism, goal orientation, and academic performance." *Anxiety, Stress, and Coping* 24, no. 2 (2011): 167-178.

2   Jason, Christopher and Lana R. Elpert. "Goal setting: effective strategies to plan for a successful career." In Habicht, Robert J. and Mangla S. Gulati, eds. *Hospital Medicine: Perspectives, Practices and Professional Development*. Cham: Springer International Publishing, 2017: 45-53.

3   Madigan, Daniel J., Joachim Stoeber, and Louis Passfield. "Perfectionism and achievement goals revisited: The 3× 2 achievement goal framework." *Psychology of Sport and Exercise* 28, no. 1 (2017): 120-124.

4   Mace, Cecil Alec. *Incentives. Some Experimental Studies*. Industrial Health Research Board Report, 72. London: Medical Research Council, 1935.

5   Ryan, Thomas Arthur and Patricia Cain Smith. *Principles of Industrial Psychology*. New York: The Ronald Press Co., 1954.

6   McClelland, David C., John W. Atkinson, Russell A. Clark, and Edgar L. Lowell. *The Achievement Motive*. New York: Appleton-Century-Crofts, 1953.

7   Weisskirch, Robert S. "Grit, self-esteem, learning strategies and attitudes and estimated and achieved course grades among college students." *Current Psychology* 7 (2016): 1-7.

8   Malvinder, Ahuja and Lata Suman. "Effect of online mastery learning on skill of acquiring knowledge in relation to self regulation and self esteem." *International Journal of Research in Social Sciences* 6, no. 10 (2016): 687-704.

9   Duckworth, Angela L. and Martin E. P. Seligman. "Self-discipline outdoes IQ in predicting academic performance of adolescents." *Psychological Science* 16, no. 12 (2005): 939-944.

10 Tangney, June P., Roy F. Baumeister, and Angie Luzio Boone. "High self-control predicts good adjustment, less pathology, better grades, and interpersonal success." *Journal of Personality* 72, no. 2 (2004): 271-324.

11 Herzberg, Frederick. "One more time: How do you motivate employees?" *Harvard Business Review* 81, no. 1 (2003): 87-96.

12 Lazenby, Scott. "How to motivate employees: What research is telling us." *Public Management* 90, no. 8 (2008): 22-25.

13 Thiedke, C. Carolyn. "What motivates staff?" *Family Practice Management* 11, no. 10 (2004): 54-56.

14 Halford, Scott G. *Activate Your Brain: How Understanding Your Brain Can Improve Your Work—And Your Life*. Austin, TX: Greenleaf Book Group, 2015.

15 Sousa, David A. *How the Brain Learns*. Thousand Oaks, CA: Corwin Press, 2011.

16 Locke, Edwin A. "Motivation through conscious goal setting." *Applied and Preventive Psychology* 5, no. 2 (1996): 117-124.

17 Locke, Edwin A. "Motivation, cognition, and action: An analysis of studies of task goals and knowledge." *Applied Psychology* 49, no. 3 (2000): 408-429.

18 Locke, Edwin A. and Gary P. Latham. "Building a practically useful theory of goal setting and task motivation: A 35-year odyssey." *American Psychologist* 57, no. 9 (2002): 705-717.

19 Locke, Edwin A. and Gary P. Latham. "New directions in goal-setting theory." *Current Directions in Psychological Science* 15, no. 5 (2006): 265-268.

20 Locke, Edwin A., Gary P. Latham, et al. *A Theory of Goal Setting and Task Performance*. Englewood Cliffs, NY: Prentice-Hall, 1990.

21 Schunk, Dale H. "Goal setting and self-efficacy during self-regulated learning." *Educational Psychologist* 25, no. 1 (1990): 71-86.

22 Zimmerman, Barry J., Albert Bandura, and Manuel Martinez-Pons. "Self-motivation for academic attainment: The role of self-efficacy beliefs and personal goal setting." *American Educational Research Journal* 29, no. 3 (1992): 663-676.

23 Richardson, Michelle, Charles Abraham, and Rod Bond. "Psychological correlates of university students' academic performance: A systematic review and meta-analysis." *Psychological Bulletin* 138, no. 2 (2012): 353-387.

24 Locke, Edwin A., Gary P. Latham, et al. *A Theory of Goal Setting and Task Performance*. Englewood Cliffs, NY: Prentice-Hall, 1990.

25 Schunk, Dale H. "Goal setting and self-efficacy during self-regulated learning." *Educational Psychologist* 25, no. 1 (1990): 71-86.

26 Latham, Gary P. and Travor C. Brown. "The effect of learning vs. outcome goals on self-efficacy, satisfaction and performance in an MBA program." *Applied Psychology* 55, no. 4 (2006): 606-623.

27 Duckworth, Angela Lee and Patrick D. Quinn. "Development and validation of the short grit scale (grit-s)." *Journal of Personality Assessment* 91, no. 2 (2009): 166-174.

28 Duckworth, Angela L., Christopher Peterson, Michael D. Matthews, and Dennis R. Kelly. "Grit: perseverance and passion for long-term goals." *Journal of Personality and Social Psychology* 92, no. 6 (2007): 1087-1101.

29 Perez, Madeline. "Obtaining academic success: Nurturing grit in students." *Journal of Interpersonal Relations, Intergroup Relations and Identity* 8 (2015): 56-63.

30 Drach-Zahavy, Anat and Miriam Erez. "Challenge versus threat effects on the goal– performance relationship." *Organizational Behavior and Human Decision Processes* 88, no. 2 (2002): 667-682.

31 Strecher, Victor J., Gerard H. Seijts, Gerjo J. Kok, Gary P. Latham, Russell Glasgow, Brenda DeVellis, Ree M. Meertens, and David W. Bulger. "Goal setting as a strategy for health behavior change." *Health Education Quarterly* 22, no. 2 (1995): 190-200.

32 Hurn, Jane, Ian Kneebone, and Mark Cropley. "Goal setting as an outcome measure: a systematic review." *Clinical Rehabilitation* 20, no. 9 (2006): 756-772.

33 Grant, Anthony M. "The impact of life coaching on goal attainment, metacognition and mental health." *Social Behavior and Personality: An International Journal* 31, no. 3 (2003): 253-263.

34 Pearson, Erin S. "Goal setting as a health behavior change strategy in overweight and obese adults: A systematic literature review examining intervention components." *Patient Education and Counseling* 87, no. 1 (2012): 32-42.

35 Shilts, Mical Kay, Marcel Horowitz, and Marilyn S. Townsend. "Goal setting as a strategy for dietary and physical activity behavior change: A review of the literature." *American Journal of Health Promotion* 19, no. 2 (2004): 81-93.

36 Bandura, Albert and Edwin A. Locke. "Negative self-efficacy and goal effects revisited." *Journal of Applied Psychology* 88 no. 1 (2003): 87-99.

37 Bandura, Albert and Dale A. Schunk. "Cultivating competence, self-efficacy, and intrinsic interest through proximal self-motivation." *Journal of Personality and Social Psychology* 41, no. 3 (1981): 586-598.

38 Gist, Marilyn E. "Self-efficacy: Implications for organizational behavior and human resource management." *Academy of Management Review* 12, no. 3 (1987): 472-485.

39 Locke, Edwin A. and Gary P. Latham. "Building a practically useful theory of goal setting and task motivation: A 35-year odyssey." *American Psychologist* 57, no. 9 (2002): 705-717.

40 Schwartz, John L. "Relationship between goal discrepancy and depression." *Journal of Consulting and Clinical Psychology* 42, no. 2 (1974): 309.

41 Campion, Michael A. and Robert G. Lord. "A control systems conceptualization of the goal-setting and changing process." *Organizational Behavior and Human Performance* 30 (1982): 265-287.

42 Hollenbeck, John R. and Charles R. Williams. "Goal importance, self-focus and the goal-setting process." *Journal of Applied Psychology* 72, no. 2 (1987): 204-211.

43 Hollenbeck, John R. and Howard J. Klein. "Goal commitment and the goal-setting process: Problems, prospects, and proposals for future research." *Journal of Applied Psychology* 72, no. 2 (1987): 212-220.

44 Latham, Gary P. and Edwin A. Locke. "New developments in and directions for goal-setting research." *European Psychologist* 12, no. 4 (2007): 290-300.

45 Ryan, Richard M. and Edward L. Deci. "Self-determination theory and the facilitation of intrinsic motivation, social development, and well-being." *American Psychologist* 55 (2000): 68-78.

46 Macan, Therese H., Comila Shahani, Robert L. Dipboye, and Amanda P. Phillips. "College students' time management: Correlations with academic performance and stress." *Journal of Educational Psychology* 82, no. 4 (1990): 760-768.

47 Misra, Ranjita and Michelle McKean. "College students' academic stress and its relation to their anxiety, time management, and leisure satisfaction." *American Journal of Health Studies* 16, no. 1 (2000): 41-51.

48 Macan, Therese Hoff. "Time management: Test of a process model." *Journal of Applied Psychology* 79, no. 3 (1994): 381-391.

49 Jex, Steve M. and Tina C. Elacqua. "Time management as a moderator of relations between stressors and employee strain." *Work & Stress* 13, no. 2 (1999): 182-191.

50 Watson, David. "Shaping by Successive Approximations." In Benjamin Jr., Ludy T. and Kathleen D. Lowman, eds. *Activities Handbook for the Teaching of Psychology*, Vol. 1. Washington, DC: American Psychological Association, 1981.

51 Zelen, Seymour L. "Goal-setting rigidity in an ambiguous situation." *Journal of Consulting Psychology* 19, no. 5 (1955): 395-399.

52 White, Paul H., Margaret M. Kjelgaard, and Stephen G. Harkins. "Testing the contribution of self-evaluation to goal-setting effects." *Journal of Personality and Social Psychology* 69, no. 1 (1995): 69-79.

53   Lochhead, Jack and Arthur Whimbey. "Teaching analytical reasoning through thinking-aloud pair problem solving." *New Directions for Teaching and Learning* 1987, no. 30 (1987): 72-93.

54   Seijts, Gerard H. and Gary P. Latham. "The effects of goal setting and group size on performance in a social dilemma." *Canadian Journal of Behavioural Science/Revue canadienne des sciences du comportement* 32, no. 2 (2000): 104-116.

55   Epstein, Joyce L. and Karen Clark Salinas. "Partnering with families and communities." *Educational Leadership* 61, no. 8 (2004): 12-18.

56   McCalley, L. T. and Cees J. H. Midden. "Energy conservation through product-integrated feedback: The roles of goal-setting and social orientation." *Journal of Economic Psychology* 23, no. 5 (2002): 589-603.

57   Smith, Ken G. and Edwin A. Locke. "Goal-setting, planning, and organizational performance: An experimental simulation." *Organizational Behavior and Human Decision Processes* 46, no. 1 (1990): 118-134.

2

FITNESS

Take care of your body. It's the only place you have to live.

— Jim Rohn

OVERVIEW

Why: Fitness is state of well-being and health as a result of proper nutrition, exercise, and rest. Practicing fitness better prepares us for the stressful rigors of our occupation and life while promoting physical, emotional, and mental well-being.

How: Develop a fitness plan. Practice the fitness plan, making modifications to better accommodate change in your lifestyle while attaining the desired fitness goal.

- Develop a fitness plan with consideration of diet, exercise, and lifestyle.
- Practice the fitness plan, tracking progress and making changes.

Identifying a measure of change after developing the goal and steps to meet the goal provides us a measure of our success. We use the subjective units of distress scale (SUDS) to help subjectively identify stress levels. Record levels before and again after as somewhere between zero (0) and ten (10), where 0 corresponds to no stress and 10 to the highest level of stress you have ever experienced. The anticipation is that the SUDS begins to decrease even after developing a goal statement and the steps to attain the goal. If your SUDS level increases, then take some time to reassess the goal statement to assure it is attainable, and reassess the steps to assure that they have been adequately defined and there are a sufficient number. After all, you want to be able to check off each step and mark progress toward reaching your goal.

Goal Setting Skill—Fitness

The visual representations can give you a better understanding of your stress and how to work through the process.

Rate the stress level you perceive

Analog SUDS	Digital SUDS	Emoji SUDS
Actually, I'm not stressed	0	
A little stressed	1–3	
Somewhat stressed	4–6	
Quite a bit stressed	7–8	
It's really bad	9	
Run and hide!!	10	

Think about what's stressing you out. What might help?

Try and identify an objective to help you do that.

Now it's time to figure out how to get there.

Write out your fitness goal statement and how you plan to get there, step-by-step.

Now get started! Don't be shy. Go for it!

Don't practice until you get it right. Practice until you can't get it wrong.

— Unknown

Have you made any progress?

Rate the stress level you perceive now

Is it lower?

Yes	No
  Congratulations!! You did it!! Now you can do this whenever you need it!	What might have gone wrong? Did you figure out all your steps? Did you actually do them all? Did you give yourself enough time? Did you enjoy your activities? Did you create enough time to exercise? Do you have an inappropriate fitness regimen? Are you impatient; did you not allow enough time to see change? Give it another try, from the beginning!

Is SUDS the only option for measuring change? Certainly not! You are encouraged to find the most appropriate measurement for your needs. The only thing that matters is that it can provide meaningful feedback with regard to change, or even transformation, resulting from applying the goal-setting process. Perhaps a scale that measures the likelihood of completing the task might be more useful. That scale might range from 0 to 10, where 0 corresponds to zero chance of completion and 10 is fully sure of completion. If you were using a likelihood-of-completion scale, then you would anticipate an increase in likelihood to complete from premeasure to postmeasure.

WHY FITNESS?

Today, less than 5% of adults in America participate in 30 minutes of exercise each day and only one in three engage in the recommended amount of weekly physical activity.[1,2] Sadly, only one in three children are physically active every day and approximately one-third of high school students play video or computer games for three or more hours on an average school day.[3,4] Research has also shown a decline in exercise among college students.[5,6] Because of our inactivity and poor eating habits, it is projected that by 2030 half of all adults in America (115 million) will be obese.[7] Medical costs for treating obesity-related illnesses is currently a $190.2 billion annual cost and rising.[8] While these statistics can be depressing, resilient people will view this data as a challenge. In fact, early pioneers in the field of resilience Suzanne Kobasa and Salvatore R. Maddi observed that resilient or hardy people have three unique characteristics: commitment, control, and challenge.[9] These three characteristics are essential in our effort to maintain an optimal level of fitness.

Physical fitness

The definition of fitness has evolved as we have evolved from hunter-gatherers to a highly industrialized society. By the mid-20th century, the definition of *fitness* had advanced from "individuals who were judged by accomplishments are fit to carry on their jobs" to include the supportive qualities of personality to complete tasks without undue fatigue or exhaustion.[10,11]

Exercise is now defined as the physical activity that is planned, structured, and repetitive with the objective of maintaining or improving physical fitness (fig. 2–1).[12,13]

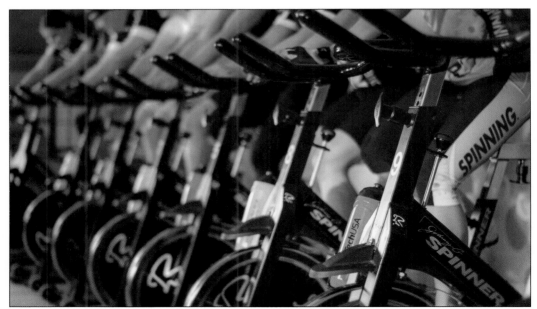

Fig. 2–1. Regular physical fitness improves health. (unsplash.com)

The concept of physical fitness emerged as both health and skill related. Presently, it is characterized by the ability to perform daily activities with vigor and with the benefit of lowering the risk of conditions associated with physical inactivity.[14] Health-related physical activity shows more desirable health outcomes across a variety of physical conditions. In general, exercise and physical activity are associated with better quality of life and health outcomes.[15] Conversely, physical inactivity is one of the most decisive risk factors for cardiovascular disease (CVD) prevalence and mortality in adults.[16]

A brief look across a lifespan argues for the importance of physical activity. And one of the best strategies for improving long-term health is to live a healthy lifestyle from an early age. Exposing children to the enjoyment of physical exercise and creating a pattern of regular physical activity is more desirable than simply promoting childhood physical fitness.[17] Active children are generally leaner, have higher peak bone masses, and display healthier cardiovascular profiles. There is also a carryover effect into adulthood with improved health and the likelihood of continuing as a more active adult.[18]

An analysis of university students from 21 countries showed that regular physical exercise was consistent with a healthy lifestyle and emotional well-being.[19] Similarly, in a survey of over 175,000 adults, the proportion of adults reporting 14 or more unhealthy physical or mental days in any given year was lower among those who attained moderate levels of physical activity compared to physically inactive adults for all age, ethnic, and sex groups.[20,21]

Even in sedentary older adults, fitness training is found to have benefits for cognition, with the largest benefits occurring for executive-control processes such as coordination, inhibition, scheduling, planning, and working memory.[22,23] There are arguments that regular exercise is associated with a lower risk for dementia.[24] Both dietary and exercise modification seem to be strong promoters of healthy aging.[25]

Physical exercise leads to improved mood, self-concept, self-esteem, and work behavior. It also appears to improve social skills and cognitive functioning.[26,27] The evidence suggests that physical activity and exercise probably alleviate some symptoms associated with mild to moderate depression and reduce the symptoms of anxiety and physiological response to stressors.[28] However, excessive physical activity may lead to overtraining and generate psychological symptoms that mimic depression.[29]

In contrast to depression, *emotional well-being* is the subjective state of wellness, happiness, and life satisfaction.[30] Well-being might be defined as a positive evaluation of one's life to include positive emotion, engagement, satisfaction, and meaning.[31,32,33]

Quality of life (QOL) is a broad, multidimensional concept that usually includes subjective evaluations of both positive and negative aspects of life that extend the definition of quality of health.[34] Health-related quality of life (HRQOL) includes aspects of life that affect perceived physical and mental health. Emotional well-being is a primary component of HRQOL and may be independently associated with the incidence of morbidity or disease and mortality.[35]

A growing body of research supports physical exercise as a lifestyle factor that might lead to increased physical and mental health throughout life.[36,37] The recommendation by the World Health Organization (WHO) is that adults who are 18–64 years old should do about 150 minutes of moderate-intensity aerobic physical activity throughout the week, or 75 minutes of vigorous-intensity aerobic physical activity throughout the week.[38] While much of the research appears to support the notion that 30 minutes of moderate leisure time physical activity per day on a regular basis may be beneficial to HRQOL, higher-intensity leisure time physical activity is associated with greater HRQOL.[39,40]

A feeble body weakens the mind.

— Jean-Jacques Rousseau

Nutritional fitness

Good nutrition promotes HRQOL by averting malnutrition, preventing dietary deficiency diseases, and promoting optimal functioning.[41] Though it may seem obvious, it is important to recognize that food security is considered an important risk factor for child health.[42] At the opposite end of the age range, older adults are at risk for poor nutrition and, therefore, frequently experience declining health-related quality of life. Put simply, nutritional risk, along with social support, appear to be significant factors associated with HRQOL.[43]

There appear to be core aspects of a healthy diet that may lower the risk of mortality outcomes for both men and women. These programs include a diet associated with the Healthy Eating Index of 2010 (HEI-2010).[44] This index is a measure of diet quality in terms of conformance with US federal dietary guidance. The HEI-2010 captures the key recommendations of the dietary guidelines and, like earlier versions, is used to assess the quality of a given dietary pattern, set of foods, or menu.[45] An index such as HEI-2010 allows measurement relative to the established index criteria and also provides an associated diet, forming the basis for meaningful research. Young women whose diets most closely met the 2010 dietary guidelines for Americans, for example, showed lower "fatness."[46]

Another healthy diet, Harvard's Healthy Eating Plate, is associated with the Alternative Healthy Eating Index, also of 2010 (AHEI-2010). Similarly, a Mediterranean diet associated with the Alternate Mediterranean Diet (aMED), and the Dietary Approaches to Stop Hypertension (DASH) Eating Plan, associated with the DASH score, consistently lower the risk of mortality. These diets tend to support consumption of higher percentages of whole grains, vegetables, fruit, and plant-based proteins.[47,48] Other dietary research suggests that high intakes of fruit, vegetables, fish, and whole grains may be associated with a reduced depression risk.[49]

Currently, the US Department of Health and Human Services has forwarded the Healthy People (HP) initiative that provides science-based, 10-year national objectives for improving health. The HP2020 iteration of the initiative measures progress toward a target attainment of more than 1,000 health-related objectives and the elimination of health disparities. Specifically, HP2020 seeks to increase life expectancy; achieve health equity; create social and physical environments that promote good health; and promote quality of life, healthy development, and healthy behaviors across all life stages.[50,51]

Don't dig your grave with your own knife and fork.

— Old English proverb

THE HOW OF FITNESS

Arguably one of the earliest and more meaningful definitions of fitness might be captured in the statement "run for your life." This obviously has evolved from having the personal resources to be able to escape danger. Run for your life can also have a different meaning. It can be seen as promoting physical and other activities to improve the sustainment and quality of life, or the lifelong run for wellness.

Wellness is often defined as a process of learning new life skills and making conscious choices to improve health and quality of life, prolong life, and achieve total well-being. WHO describes these lifestyle changes as occurring across seven dimensions:[52,53]

- Social
- Physical
- Emotional
- Career
- Intellectual
- Environmental
- Spiritual

Physical wellness is the process of making choices to create strong bodies with consideration of exercise, nutrition, rest and sleep, responsible sexual choices, and management of stress, injury, and illness.[54] The focus of the fitness skill is that of physical wellness (fig. 2–2).

Rest and sleep skills are addressed in chapter 3.

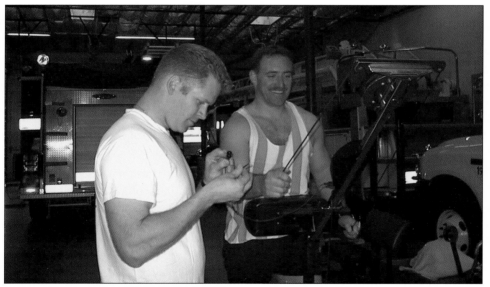

Fig. 2–2. Physical wellness includes exercise. (Courtesy of Mike Grill.)

Exercise

An essential aspect of physical wellness is that of exercise. A foundational physical fitness plan might begin with consideration of the 2008 Physical Activity Guidelines for Americans. The associated research on the benefits of physical activity is summarized in the following list:[55]

- Regular physical activity reduces the risk of many adverse health outcomes.
- Some physical activity is better than none.

- For most health outcomes, additional benefits occur as the amount of physical activity increases through higher intensity, greater frequency, and/or longer duration.

- Most health benefits occur with at least 150 minutes a week of moderate-intensity physical activity, such as brisk walking. Additional benefits occur with more physical activity.

- Both aerobic (endurance) and muscle-strengthening (resistance) physical activity are beneficial. When combined, the benefits are even better.

- Health benefits occur for children and adolescents, young and middle-aged adults, and older adults (although the exercise process may differ between groups).

- The health benefits of physical activity also occur for people with disabilities, of course.

- The benefits of physical activity far outweigh the possibility of adverse outcomes.

The basis of the Physical Activity Guidelines for Americans program is aerobic physical activity. Adults are to do 2½ hours (150 minutes) of moderate-intensity or 1¼ hours (75 minutes) of vigorous-intensity aerobic physical activity each week. Another option is to perform an equivalent combination of moderate- and vigorous-intensity aerobic physical activity. Such activity is performed in episodes of at least 10 minutes, preferably spread throughout the week. Additional health benefits may be provided by increasing activity to 5 hours of moderate-intensity or 2½ hours of vigorous-intensity aerobic physical activity each week. Again, an equivalent combination of both is as effective, if not more so. Muscle-strengthening activities that involve all the major muscle groups, on two or more days per week, is encouraged. Of the movement styles, current recommendations focus on movements incorporating action that involves multiple joints. Research is evolving indicating that such multi-joint movements tend to produce good results while reducing the injuries that can occur with single-joint movements.

As much as possible, older adults (65 and older) should adhere to the recommendation of 2½ hours of moderate-intensity aerobic physical activity a week. But let's be realistic. If chronic conditions exist, then the adult should be as physically active as abilities and conditions allow. It is vital that you find a level of effort based on your understanding of how any personal chronic conditions affect your abilities. If you don't, the likelihood of frustration, pain, or even injury will short-circuit all your good intentions. Finally, you should include exercises that maintain or improve your balance to reduce your risk of falling.

Children and adolescents, ages 6 to 17, should exercise 60 or more minutes a day performing moderate- or vigorous-intensity aerobic physical activity, with vigorous-intensity physical activity at least three days a week. A part of daily physical activity should include muscle strengthening at least three days of the week. Examples of muscle-strengthening activities include unstructured exercise, such as playing on playground equipment, climbing trees, and playing tug-of-war and structured exercise, such as lifting weights or working with resistance bands. Additionally, part of the daily physical activity should include bone-strengthening at least three days of the week. Common bone-strengthening activities (also referred to as impact activities) include running, jumping rope, and playing games such as basketball, tennis, and hopscotch.[56]

How are the guidelines translated into a meaningful exercise program? One method might be to consider your general intentions, preferences, and limitations.[57] However, at the core, you will need to begin to focus more mindfully on why you want to improve your fitness. Once you have done this, consider the following:

■ What are your goals? Are your interests health, fitness, or performance related?

_____

_____

_____

_____

■ What do you enjoy? Do you prefer team or solitary activities?

_____

_____

_____

_____

■ What are your time limits? How much time can you devote?

_____

_____

_____

_____

■ What gear do you need? What is your budget?

_____

_____

_____

_____

How do we better define these guidelines into something more specific and measurable? We can track how much activity is occurring across the course of a week through the use of the metabolic equivalent of task (MET), or metabolic equivalent, which is a physiological measure describing the energy used for physical activity. More specifically, the MET is the ratio of the rate of energy (calories) expended during an activity to the rate of energy expended at rest. One MET is the energy equivalent expended by an individual while at rest. A 3 MET activity, for example, expends three times the energy used by the body at rest. If you were to do an activity of 3 METs intensity for 20 minutes, you would have done 3 × 20 = 60 MET minutes of physical activity. A range from 500 to 1,000 MET minutes per week is considered the amount of physical activity necessary to produce meaningful health benefits. But, recognize that the higher the minutes, the more beneficial the effect.[58] Thus, the specific intensity of an aerobic exercise factors into the calculation.

- Light-intensity activities are defined as 1.1 to 2.9 METs.
- Moderate-intensity activities are defined as 3.0 to 5.9 METs.

- For example, walking at 3.0 miles per hour requires 3.3 METs of energy expenditure and is therefore considered a moderate-intensity activity.

- Vigorous-intensity activities are defined as 6.0 METs or higher. For example, running at 10 minutes per mile is a 10 MET activity and is therefore classified as vigorous intensity.

There are associated MET values for many common exercises:

Activity	Equivalent MET
Gardening	2.5
Walking, moderate pace	3.5
Swimming	6.0
Jogging	7.0
General bicycling	7.5

An extensive variety of information is available online, including the Compendium of Physical Activities, to find the MET value for different activities as well as more detailed information on variations of exercises.[59]

Beyond the MET value, though, you may be interested in the number of calories you are burning. To convert your body weight from pounds to kilograms, divide by 2.2. From that value you can calculate calories per minute:

$$(\text{MET value} \times 3.5 \times \text{weight in kg})/200 = \text{calories burned per minute}$$

For example, consider a 150 lb (68 kg) person who runs for 30 minutes at a 6 mph pace (10 METs). (10 METs × 3.5 × 68 kg)/200 = 2,380/200 = 11.9 calories burned per minute. Then, as above, 11.9 × 30 min = 357 calories burned per 30-minute run.

For health benefits for most adults, the national guidelines suggest burning 1,000 calories per week. For weight loss and even greater health benefits, an expenditure of 2,000 calories per week is suggested.[60,61]

Need some motivation? Some research suggests we can calculate our fitness age based on our peak oxygen intake (VO_2), which is correlated to lifespan. VO_2 and fitness age can be calculated without a treadmill by using several measurements that include waist size, resting heart rate, age, sex, and frequency and intensity of exercise.[62] An online fitness calculator to determine fitness age can be found on the Norwegian University of Science and Technology's (NTNU) website.[63]

The wise man should consider that health is the greatest of human blessings.
Let food be your medicine.

— Hippocrates

Nutrition

Another aspect of physical wellness is that of nutrition. A foundational dietary plan might begin with a look at several diets that may lower the risk of mortality (fig. 2–3).[64]

HEI-2010 and the 2015–2020 Dietary Guidelines for Americans. A diet adhering to HEI-2010 captures the key recommendations of the 2010 Dietary Guidelines and can be used to assess the quality of a menu. The 2015–2020 Dietary Guidelines for Americans is a revision to the 2010 guidelines and reflects research that demonstrates eating patterns and physical activity can help people achieve and maintain good health and reduce the risk of chronic disease throughout their lifespan.

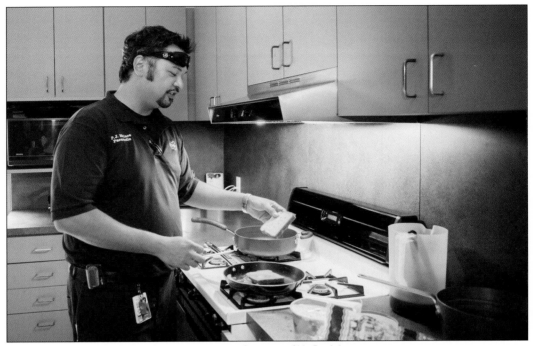

Fig. 2–3. Dieting can reduce your risk of mortality. (Courtesy of Vu Banh.)

Several terms used throughout the guidelines provide an orientation to the approach. A dietary pattern or *eating pattern* describes a customary way of eating or a combination of foods recommended for consumption. *Nutrient-dense* describes foods and beverages that provide vitamins, minerals, and other substances that contribute to adequate nutrient intakes or may have positive health effects, with little or no solid fats, added sugars, refined starches, or sodium. This includes all vegetables, fruits, whole grains, seafood, eggs, beans and peas, unsalted nuts and seeds, fat-free and low-fat dairy products, and lean meats and poultry. *Variety* describes an assortment of foods and beverages across and within all food groups and subgroups selected to fulfill the recommended amounts without exceeding the limits for calories and other dietary components. The term *shift* is used to emphasize the need to make substitutions, that is, choose nutrient-dense foods and beverages in place of less healthy choices rather than increasing the overall intake. This focus on shifts in eating patterns is intended to align current dietary intake with recommendations and highlight multiple strategies across all segments of society to promote healthy eating and physical activity behaviors.[65,66]

There are five guidelines regarding eating patterns:

- Follow a healthy eating pattern across the lifespan. Choose a healthy eating pattern at an appropriate calorie level to help achieve and maintain a healthy body weight, support nutrient adequacy, and reduce the risk of chronic disease.

- Focus on variety, nutrient density, and amount. Choose a variety of nutrient-dense foods across and within all food groups in recommended amounts.

- Limit calories from added sugars and saturated fats and reduce sodium intake. Follow an eating pattern low in added sugars, saturated fats, and sodium. Cut back on foods and beverages higher in these components to amounts that fit within healthy eating patterns.

- Shift to healthier food and beverage choices (fig. 2–4). Choose nutrient-dense foods and beverages across and within all food groups in place of less healthy choices. Consider cultural and personal preferences to make these shifts easier to accomplish and maintain.

- Support healthy eating patterns for all. Everyone has a role in helping create and support healthy eating patterns. These social determinants of health and the economics of public health and prevention are similarly echoed in a global manner by the World Health Organization.[67]

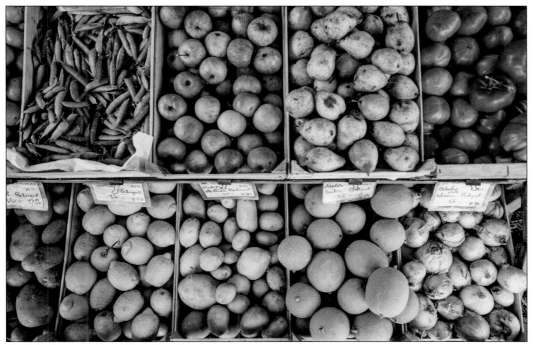

Fig. 2–4. Eating the right foods contributes to good health. (unsplash.com)

Additionally, the following recommendations for healthy eating patterns should be applied in their entirety due to the interconnected relationship of each dietary component:

- A healthy eating pattern accounts for all foods and beverages within an appropriate calorie level.

- A healthy eating pattern includes a variety of vegetables from all of the subgroups and the following:

  - Dark-green, red, and orange vegetables

  - Legumes (beans and peas), starchy and other

  - Fruits, especially whole fruits

  - Grains, at least half of which are whole grains

- – Fat-free or low-fat dairy, including milk, yogurt, cheese, and/or fortified soy beverages

- – A variety of protein foods, including seafood, lean meats and poultry, eggs, legumes, nuts, seeds, and soy products

- – Oils

- A healthy eating pattern limits saturated fats and trans fats, added sugars, and sodium.

There are recommended numerical limits in calories to help individuals achieve healthy eating patterns based on their desired weight and lifestyle. These include consuming less than 10% of calories per day from added sugars, less than 10% of calories per day from saturated fats, less than 2,300 milligrams (mg) per day of sodium, and if alcohol is consumed, it should be consumed in moderation of one drink per day for females and two for males.

So where does one begin constructing a healthy diet in accordance with these guidelines? While the entire guidelines are downloadable, they can also be implemented by using online tools as MyPlate, which provides the opportunity to establish personal baseline measures, create a healthy diet, and track fitness-related results.[68] A basic 2,000-calorie daily menu might look like the following one:[69]

Breakfast	Morning snack	Lunch	Afternoon snack	Dinner
1 ounce grains	1 ounce grains	2 ounces grains	½ cup vegetables	2 ounces grains
½ cup fruits	1 cup fruits	1 cup vegetables	½ cup dairy	1 cup vegetables
½ cup dairy		½ cup fruits		1 cup dairy
		1 cup dairy		3 ounces protein foods
		2½ ounces protein foods		

The menu presumes a 2,000-calorie daily plan. Based on variables such as activity, gender, age, height, and weight, an individual can calculate the appropriate baseline caloric intake for more accurately determining meal and snack quantities. We want to regulate the total amount of energy, which the body receives through food intake, and balance this with the total amount of energy that the body expends.

Food energy comes into the body in the form of solids and fluids. The body expends energy through its process of maintaining life, its digestion and absorption of food, and its physical activity. Overall, we are seeking an energy balance, where energy balance is the difference between the number of calories you eat (intake) and the number of calories you burn (output).

Side note: The term *calorie* generally refers to the kilogram calorie. The convention of using the capital C for the kilogram calorie and the lowercase c for the gram calorie is advocated by some, but is not universally followed (1,000 calories = 1 kilocalorie (kcal) = 1 Calorie).

For men, the following calculation can be used to obtain your basal metabolic rate (BMR) in kcal/day:

$$66 + (6.23 \times \text{weight in pounds}) + (12.7 \times \text{height in inches}) - (6.8 \times \text{age in years}) \text{ or}$$
$$66 + (13.75 \times \text{weight in kg}) + (5 \times \text{height in cm}) - (6.8 \times \text{age in years})$$

For example, a 27-year-old male who is 5'11" (71") tall and weighs 190 pounds is calculated as follows:

$$66 + (6.23 \times 190) + (12.7 \times 71) - (6.8 \times 27) = 66 + 1,184 + 902 - 184 = 1,968 \text{ kcal/day}$$

For women, this calculation can be used to approximate the BMR:

$$655 + (4.35 \times \text{weight in pounds}) + (4.7 \times \text{height in inches}) - (4.7 \times \text{age in years}) \text{ or}$$
$$655 + (9.56 \times \text{weight in kg}) + (1.8 \times \text{height in cm}) - (4.7 \times \text{age in years})$$

For example, a 27-year-old female who is 5'4" (64") tall and weighs 120 pounds is calculated as follows:

$$655 + (4.35 \times 120) + (4.7 \times 64) - (4.7 \times 27) = 655 + 522 + 301 - 127 = 1{,}351 \text{ kcal/day}$$

Once the BMR is determined, an activity estimate is identified:

Characterization	Activities	Factor
Very light:	Sitting, standing, driving, computer work	1.2
Light:	Walking, light stretching, woodworking	1.4
Moderate:	Jogging, dancing, swimming, biking	1.6
Strenuous:	Running, soccer, rowing, digging, carrying	1.9

The Harris-Benedict equation can be used to estimate the daily caloric requirement by multiplying the BMR times the activity factor. The obtained value indicates your energy needs or estimated energy requirement (EER), with the number of calories of energy you need per day in order to meet your expected body needs.

$$\text{EER} = \text{BMR} \times \text{activity factor}$$

For example, consider again the 27-year-old male who is 5'11" tall and weighs 190 pounds. His BMR is determined to be 1,968 cal. Then, if we assume his activity factor is 1.4:

$$\text{EER} = 1{,}968 \times 1.4 \text{ or } 2{,}755 \text{ kcal/day}$$

Another useful baseline measure is to obtain an approximation of one's body composition. The body mass index (BMI) provides an estimate of whether one's weight is in accordance with one's height. BMI has often been associated with stress-related research. Those with a very low BMI tend to lose weight when stressed and, conversely, those with a high BMI tend to gain weight when stressed.[70,71,72]

$$\text{BMI} = \text{body weight in pounds} \times 705 / \text{height in inches squared}$$

Work-related stress should also be taken into account as having potential impact on weight gain and loss.[73]

Metabolic syndrome is the name for a group of risk factors that raises the likelihood for heart disease and other health problems such as cancer and diabetes. Characteristics of the metabolic syndrome include abdominal obesity and high blood pressure.[74,75,76]

Alternatively, using an online tool such as MyPlate Super Tracker will automatically calculate your caloric intake and further allow you to set goals such as establishing a preferred body weight and tracking your results as you progress to your goal. Goal setting shows great promise as a tool that can be incorporated into weight reduction programs by health care professionals and researchers.[77]

AHEI-2010 and Harvard's Healthy Eating Plate. The Harvard School of Public Health developed the Alternate Healthy Eating Index (AHEI) with a scoring system similar to the USDA's index. AHEI assesses 11 components:

- Dairy products

- Vegetables
- Fruit
- Cholesterol
- Fat
- Sodium
- Alcohol
- Multivitamins
- Nuts and seeds
- Bread and grains
- Fish, poultry, and meat

The Healthy Eating Plate template serves as a concise and functional guide for creating high quality meals (fig. 2–5). Based on the plate template, half of your plate is vegetables and fruits. You are encouraged to omit potatoes, but otherwise aim for color and variety. A quarter of your plate should be whole and intact grains to include whole wheat, barley, wheat berries, quinoa, oats, brown rice, and foods made with them such as whole wheat pasta. A quarter of your plate should be protein to include fish, chicken, beans, and nuts and foods made with them such as salads. Limit red meat, and avoid processed meats such as bacon and sausage. Healthy plant oils can be used in moderation. Consider olive, canola, soy, corn, sunflower, peanut, and other oils, but avoid partially hydrogenated oils containing trans fats. Drink water, coffee, or tea. Omit sugary drinks, and limit juice to one small glass per day and milk and dairy products to one to two servings per day. Finally, you are encouraged to be active for health and weight control.[78,79,80]

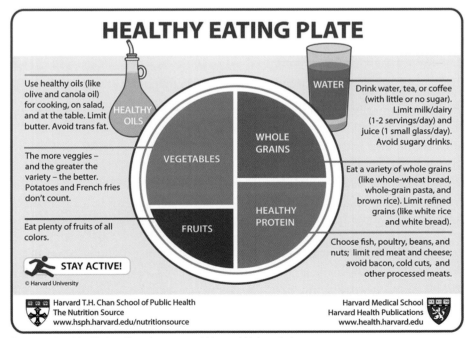

Fig. 2–5. Healthy Eating Plate (courtesy of Harvard University)

The Mediterranean diet and aMED. The Mediterranean diet (MED) and the alternate Mediterranean diet (aMED) are conformity scales for measuring characteristics of a Mediterranean and modified Mediterranean diet. There are variations to the diet, with the healthier variants sharing common characteristics, such as being higher in fresh fruits, root and green vegetables, whole grains, and fish that is rich in omega-3 fatty acids, but being much lower in red meat. The Mediterranean diets also substitute low- or nonfat dairy products for high-fat, and further substitute olive oil, nuts, or margarines blended with rapeseed or flaxseed oils for butter and fats:[81]

Monthly	Weekly	Daily	
Meat	Sweets	Cheese, yogurt	Rice
	Eggs	Olive oil	Couscous
	Poultry	Fruits	Barley
	Fish	Beans, legumes, and nuts	Other whole grains and potatoes
		Whole-grain bread	Daily physical activity
		Pasta	

A sample one-day, 2,000 or lower calorie diet might appear much like the following:

Breakfast	One slice of whole-grain bread spread with one tablespoon of nut butter or two ounces of avocado
	One cup of sliced strawberries with one cup of fruit yogurt
Lunch	Tossed salad with one-half cup of beans and one-half ounce of nuts dressed with one tablespoon of olive oil with vinegar or lemon juice and herbs
Dinner	Fish baked or grilled, with olive oil, three ounces cooked (about four ounces raw)
	Half-plate serving of vegetables
	One-half cup of whole grain such as brown rice
Snacks	One cup of plain Greek yogurt with one-half cup of blueberries, or
	One ounce or handful of nuts plus a plate of raw vegetables, or
	Two tablespoons hummus with five whole-grain crackers and a cup of vegetables

There is strong evidence for a beneficial effect of the Mediterranean dietary patterns on risk of death from all causes, including deaths due to cardiovascular disease and cancer, in a US population.[82] Similarly, the Mediterranean diet, modified so as to apply across nine European countries, was associated with increased survival among older people.[83]

DASH and the DASH eating plan. The DASH diet is a lifelong approach to healthy eating that is designed primarily to treat or prevent hypertension but is also consistent with dietary recommendations to help prevent osteoporosis, cancer, heart disease, stroke, and diabetes.[84]

Fruits: Eat four to five servings per day of apples, bananas, berries, oranges, pineapple, peaches, pears, grapes, melons, raisins, or dried apricots. Limit sweets and added sugars to five or less servings per week.

Vegetables: Include four to five servings per day of asparagus, broccoli, carrots, collards, green beans, green peas, kale, lettuce, lima beans, potatoes, spinach, squash, sweet potatoes, or tomatoes.

Grains: Eat six to eight servings per day of whole wheat bread, whole wheat pasta, English muffin, pita, bagel, cereals, grits, oatmeal, quinoa, brown rice, unsalted pretzels, or popcorn.

Protein (dairy, meat, nuts, seeds, legumes): Limit dairy to two to three servings per day of fat-free or low-fat milk, buttermilk, cheese, or yogurt. Eat six or less servings per day of broiled, roasted, or poached fish, lean meats, or poultry. Limit nuts, seeds, and legumes such as almonds, hazelnuts, peanuts, walnuts, sunflower seeds, peanut butter, kidney beans, lentils, and split peas to four to five servings per week.

Fats and oils: Include two to three servings per day of canola, corn, olive, or safflower oils (one teaspoon), soft margarine (one teaspoon), low-fat mayonnaise (one tablespoon), or light salad dressing (two tablespoons).

There are two versions of the diet, where the standard DASH diet allows up to 2,300 mg and the lower sodium diet up to 1,500 mg of sodium a day. The diet tends to be low in saturated fat and cholesterol and therefore encourages vegetables, fruits, and low-fat dairy foods with moderate amounts of whole grains, fish, poultry, and nuts:[85]

- Eat vegetables, fruits, and whole grains.
- Include fat-free or low-fat dairy products, fish, poultry, beans, nuts, and vegetable oils.
- Limit foods that are high in saturated fat, such as fatty meats, full-fat dairy products, and tropical oils such as coconut, palm kernel, and palm oils.
- Avoid sugary beverages and sweets.

Because of the emphasis on lowering blood pressure, the foods are lower in sodium but higher in potassium, magnesium, and calcium. A sample one-day 2,000-calorie diet would assume low salt and might appear much like the following:[86]

Breakfast	One whole wheat bagel with two tablespoons peanut butter (no salt added) One medium orange One cup fat-free milk Decaffeinated coffee
Lunch	Spinach salad made with four cups of fresh spinach leaves, sliced pear, one-half cup canned mandarin orange sections, one-third cup slivered almonds, and two tablespoons red wine vinaigrette Twelve reduced-sodium wheat crackers One cup fat-free milk
Dinner	Herb-crusted baked cod, three ounces cooked (about four ounces raw) One-half cup brown rice pilaf with vegetables One-half cup fresh green beans, steamed One small sourdough roll Two teaspoons olive oil One cup fresh berries with chopped mint Herbal iced tea
Snack (anytime)	One cup fat-free, low-calorie yogurt Four vanilla wafers

A more accurate caloric intake can be calculated by factors such as activity level, age, gender, height, and weight. The number of servings is determined based on the number of calories you are allowed each day. The caloric intake can be adjusted upward to gain weight or downward to lose weight. If you intend to lose weight, it is typically desirable to include exercise as a part of your plan.

Table 2–1, adapted from the National Institute of Health's DASH Eating Plan, can be used to determine servings and serving sizes based on the nearest caloric grouping:[87]

Table 2–1. DASH eating plan

DASH Eating Plan Caloric Servings Per Day Reference				
Food group	**1,600**	**2,000**	**2,600**	**Serving sizes**
Grains	6	6–8	10–11	1 slice bread; 1 oz. cereal; 1/2 cup cooked rice, pasta, or cereal
Vegetables	3–4	4–5	5–6	1 cup raw leafy vegetable, 1/2 cup raw or cooked vegetable, 1/2 cup vegetable juice
Fruits	4	4–5	5–6	1 medium fruit; 1/4 cup dried fruit; 1/2 cup fresh, frozen, or canned fruit; 1/2 cup juice
Fat-free or low-fat milk products	2–3	2–3	3	1 cup milk or yogurt, 11/2 oz. cheese
Lean meats, poultry, and fish	3–6	≤6	6	1 oz. cooked meats, poultry, or fish; 1 egg
Nuts, seeds, and legumes	3 per week	4–5 per week	1	1/3 cup nuts, 2 Tbsp peanut butter, 2 Tbsp seeds, 1/2 cup cooked legumes
Fats and oils	2	2–3	3	1 tsp soft margarine, 1 tsp vegetable oil, 1 Tbsp mayonnaise, 2 Tbsp salad dressing
Sweets and sugars	0	≤5	<2	1 Tbsp sugar, 1 Tbsp jelly or jam, 1/2 cup sorbet or gelatin, 1 cup lemonade

The DASH diet, with a low sodium level, has demonstrated a significant reduction of systolic blood pressure of around 7 mmHg lower in people without hypertension, and around 11 mmHg lower in people with hypertension.[88,89] Even larger blood pressure reductions occur for overweight or obese persons with the addition of exercise and weight loss to the DASH diet.[90,91]

Gluttony is an emotional escape, a sign something is eating us.

— Peter De Vries

Example of fitness

I need to get into better shape. I have decided to take a look at my diet and exercise and come up with a plan that suits my lifestyle yet keeps me in shape (fig. 2–6). This equates to a lot of change for me and my SUDS is starting about 4. I'm not really sure which diet plan to use so my plan is try four different plans: MyPlate, Healthy Plate, Mediterranean, and DASH. I'll first use an online calculator to determine my recommended caloric intake using gender, height, weight, and age. The calorie value will be used to determine quantity portions for the diet plans. This will better assure I have a good baseline from which to compare diet plans. I will try each diet plan for a week using an online source of daily menus. I will then determine which dietary plan appears to work best for me.

My exercise plan is a simple cardiac type of workout of about 30 minutes per day, five days per week. I am fairly sure I can maintain this regimen. During the four-week period I am testing the diet plans, I will also keep a log of my exercise. I intend to rotate walking, jogging, and maybe biking on the weekend. After completing this goal-setting phase of the fitness process, my SUDS is down to a 3.

I have tried the four diet plans and continued exercising over the past month. Despite all of the change, I am feeling better and more in control. My SUDS is down to a 2.

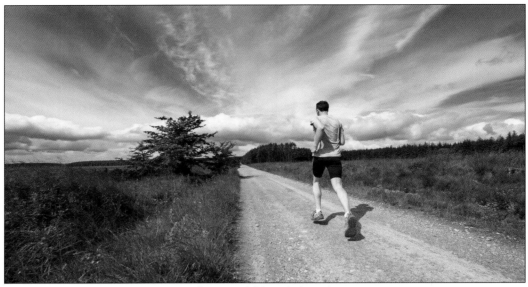

Fig. 2–6. Do you have an exercise plan or fitness goals? (unsplash.com)

Fitness

Identify SUDS (0–10) SUDS: 4

Create fitness plan:

> Nutritional goal: Try each of the four diet plans for one week.
>
> > Step 1: Calculate caloric intake applying to plans.
> >
> > Step 2: Use MyPlate online for one-week plan.
> >
> > Step 3: Use online sources for one week of Healthy Plate.
> >
> > Step 4: Use online sources for one week of Mediterranean diet.
> >
> > Step 5: Use online resources for one week of DASH diet.
>
> Exercise goal: Develop an exercise plan of 2 hours and 30 minutes a week of moderate intensity.
>
> > Step 1: Identify 30 minutes per day for five days per week exercise plan.
> >
> > Step 2: Rotate walking, jogging, and biking days.

Identify SUDS (0–10) SUDS: 3

> SUDS lower? *Yes*

Practice fitness:

> Goal: Complete a one-week diet for each of the four plans and pick the one that works best.
>
> > Step 1: Maintain a basic daily log of what worked and what didn't.
>
> Goal: Develop an exercise plan of 2 hours and 30 minutes a week of moderate intensity.
>
> > Step 1: Maintain a progress log for one month.

SUDS: 2

SUDS lower? *Yes*

> *By writing out my fitness goals I was able to clarify my thinking and establish a series of steps that allowed me to establish a healthy diet plan and an exercise plan I could maintain. I continue to use both the diet and exercise plans to provide me a sense of being able to persist while lowering my level of stress.*

Exercise to stimulate, not to annihilate. The world wasn't formed in a day, and neither were we. Set small goals and build upon them.

— Lee Haney

INTERNALIZE FITNESS

Recall, in as much detail as possible, a past personal experience where you practiced fitness as exercise, diet, or both. Given that fitness experience, translate it to the fitness skill. If you prefer, consider writing about your fitness experience as a brief story and build in the fitness skill. Work on this process individually or in collaboration (fig. 2–6).

Checklist for internalizing fitness

A *scoring rubric* is intended to communicate expectations of quality regarding a particular task. The rubric functions as an aid or checklist for task completion and provides a basis for self-evaluation, reflection, and comparable peer review.

Consider using the following checklist as a rubric or map for completing this leg of your journey.

Checklist for Internalizing Fitness

Think back. Is there a past situation you really thought about after it was all over?

Identify, as best you can recall, the event.

Did you see this as an adversity?   Why?

Did you see this as an opportunity?   Why?

When you started to review your results, try to remember your baseline SUDS.

How did this situation fit with what you had thought about before?

Did thinking about this change your SUDS?   Why?

Identify, as best you can recall, the following:

What fitness plan did you try?

How did you practice it?

Did you enjoy your choice?

How did you do?

After you reviewed these results, try to remember your resulting SUDS.

Do you think you might have used any of our other skills?   Which ones?

Now let's think about whether all this helped.

Did this process make your impression of the event more manageable?   How?

Did this process make your impression of the event more compelling?   How?

Can you think of anything you might change in this skill to make it more personally useful?

How about the future? Do you think you will be able to put your results to the test?

If writing this as narrative, in a story format, the above guide can be used as an example of how this might be done. The guide blends the bulleted rubric elements into the narrative.

Remember that writing can be a powerful tool in clarifying, recalling, and integrating the skill into your life.

_____

_____

_____

_____

He that takes medicine and neglects diet, wastes the skill of the physician.

— Chinese proverb

EXTERNALIZE: APPLY FITNESS AS A GROUP

Another process that can be of aid in small group discussions is to assign roles. For example, one person can be the facilitator assuring that all rubric items are being answered, another person can be the note taker, and yet another can be the timekeeper and summarizer.

Case study: "Well, he got accepted into his college of choice, but he is stressed about succeeding," your sister says.

"Anything I can do?" you respond.

Your sister goes on to explain that she has read where a good diet and exercise program is likely to benefit her son academically, as well as his self-esteem.[92,93] She has decided to work with him on finding a diet plan he can stick to and perhaps a simple exercise plan for while he is away at school.

"I think it would be great if you could work with us on this program. He does look up to you," she says.

How might you respond this situation? Your goal is to use fitness and any other appropriate skills to develop a potential solution.

We do not stop exercising because we grow old;
we grow old because we stop exercising.

— Dr. Kenneth Cooper

PRACTICE FITNESS

You have applied the new skill format to an instance that had occurred in your past. You have also applied the skill as a group in problem-based learning. Now, consider how you would best apply the fitness skill to a current event you are facing. Practicing the skill provides an opportunity to reflect on prior learning and make the skill more personally memorable.

Developing *automaticity*, or a habit, typically requires a period of weeks but depends upon the complexity of the task. Developing the habit of exercising, for example, may require some time before it feels normal, so allow yourself some time to test your fitness plan. Keeping a fitness or exercise log can be helpful for monitoring progress and developing a sense of automaticity.

Checklist for Practicing Fitness

Thinking carefully, what do you see as the issue(s) and need(s) that need to be addressed?

Identify, as best you can, the dilemma.

    What are your fitness goals?

    Did you see this as an adversity?   Why?

    Did you see this as an opportunity?   Why?

When you started to review your plans, what is your baseline SUDS?

    How does this situation fit with what you had thought about before?

    Did thinking about this change your SUDS?   Why?

Now, the what, where, and how.

    What fitness plan will you try?

    How will you practice it?

    How long will you commit?

After you reviewed these steps, what is your resulting SUDS?

    Do you think you might use any of our other skills (in particular, time management)?
                                                                    Which ones?

Now let's think about whether all this helps.

    Will tracking your exercise progress generate greater incentive to continue?

    Will tracking your exercise provide better feedback?

    Did this process make your impression of the event more manageable?   How?

    Did this process make your impression of the event more compelling?   How?

Can you think of anything you might change in this skill to make it more personally useful?

How about the future? Do you think you will be able to put your results to the test?

If writing this as narrative, in a story format, the above guide can be used as an example of how this might be organized.

_____

_____

_____

_____

Fitness. If it came in a bottle, everybody would have a great body.

— Cher

APPLY FITNESS TO YOUR COMMUNITY

Community can be defined as any group of people living, working, or sharing common interests such as a family, team, work group, or perhaps a neighborhood. You have applied the fitness skill to yourself and to another person as a small group exercise. Think about how you can apply this skill into your family. Do you and your partner go for walks? How much time do you engage with others in your community (or your children) in fitness activities? These can include taking opportunities to encourage healthy eating habits by having children involved in shopping for and preparing meals. Sadly, only about one in five homes have parks within a half-mile, and about the same number have a fitness or recreation center within that distance.[94] And only six states (Illinois, Hawaii, Massachusetts, Mississippi, New York, and Vermont) require physical education in every grade, K–12.[95] Approach your community leaders to increase the number of parks and playgrounds in your communities. Communities are finding creative ways to improve eating habits and improve their local economies.[96,97] If possible, consider creating community gardens and supporting local farmers as ways of applying this skill to your larger community.

Checklist for Applying Fitness to Your Community

Can you think of a community situation that might benefit from the fitness skill?

Thinking carefully, what do you see as the issue(s) and need(s) that need to be addressed?

Identify, as best you can, the dilemma.

What are your proposed community fitness goals?

Do you see this as an adversity?   Why?

Do you see this as an opportunity?   Why?

When you start to review these plans, what is your baseline SUDS?

How does this situation fit with what you had thought about before?

Does thinking about this change your SUDS?   Why?

Now, the what, where, and how.

What fitness plan will you suggest?

How will you expect the community to practice it?

How long will you suggest they commit?

After you reviewed these steps, what is your resulting SUDS.

Do you think you might suggest using any of our other skills?

In particular, time management?

Any others?

Now let's think about whether all this will be helpful to the community.

Will tracking their exercise progress generate greater incentive to continue?

Will tracking their exercising provide better feedback?

Does this process make your impression of the event more manageable?   How?

Does this process make your impression of the event more compelling?   How?

How do you think you'll do as a mentor?

Can you think of anything you might change in this skill to make it more useful?

How about the future? Do you think you will be able to put your results to the test?

If writing this as narrative, in a story format, the above guide can be used as an example of how this might be organized.

_____
_____
_____
_____

Practice puts brains in your muscles.

— Sam Snead

REMEMBERING FITNESS

We have examined and applied the new fitness skill to others and ourselves. Take the opportunity now to reflect on the skill and associate some key words or phrases that help to succinctly define the skill using your own words. When you have completed this process, compare these key words and phrases with the person or persons with whom you are working. Discuss and decide if you wish to alter any of your reflective key words or phrases. What have you learned through this process?

_____
_____
_____

Every morning in Africa, a gazelle wakes up. It knows it must outrun the fastest lion or it will be killed. Every morning in Africa, a lion wakes up. It knows it must run faster than the slowest gazelle or it will starve. It doesn't matter whether you're a lion or gazelle; when the sun comes up, you'd better be running.

— Author unknown

NOTES

1   US Department of Agriculture. *Dietary Guidelines for Americans, 2010-2020.* Available at http://www.cnpp.usda.gov/dietaryguidelines.htm.

2   US Department of Health and Human Services. *Healthy People 2010.* Available at http://www.cdc.gov/nchs/healthy_people/hp2010.htm.

3   National Association for Sport and Physical Education. *The Fitness Equation: Physical Activity + Balanced Diet = Fit Kids.* Reston, VA: National Association for Sport and Physical Education, 1999.

4   Centers for Disease Control and Prevention. "Youth Risk Behavior Surveillance—United States, 2011." *Morbidity and Mortality Weekly Report* (MMWR) 61, no. SS-66104 (2012): 1-168. Available at http://www.cdc.gov/mmwr/preview/mmwrhtml/ss6104a1.htm.

5   Ebben, William and Laura Brudzynski. "Motivations and barriers to exercise among college students." *Journal of Exercise Physiology Online* 11, no. 5 (2008): 1-11.

6   Wallace, Lorraine Silver, Janet Buckworth, Timothy E. Kirby, and W. Michael Sherman. "Characteristics of exercise behavior among college students: Application of social cognitive theory to predicting stage of change." *Preventive Medicine* 31, no. 5 (2000): 494-505.

7   Glickman, Dan, Lynn Parker, Leslie J. Sim, Heather Del Valle Cook, and Emily Ann Miller, eds. *Accelerating Progress in Obesity Prevention: Solving the Weight of the Nation.* Washington, DC: National Academies Press, 2012.

8   Wang, Y. Claire, Klim McPherson, Tim Marsh, Steven L. Gortmaker, and Martin Brown. "Health and economic burden of the projected obesity trends in the USA and the UK." *The Lancet* 378, no. 9793 (2011): 815-825.

9   Kobasa, Suzanne C., Salvatore R. Maddi, and Stephen Kahn. "Hardiness and health: A prospective study." *Journal of Personality and Social Psychology* 42, no. 1 (1982): 168-177.

10   Penrose, L. S. "The meaning of fitness in human populations." *Annals of Eugenics* 14, no. 1 (1947): 301-304.

11   Darling, Robert C., Ludwig W. Eichna, Clark W. Heath, and Harold G. Wolff. "Physical fitness: Report of the subcommittee of the Baruch committee on physical medicine." *Journal of the American Medical Association* 136, no. 11 (1948): 764-767.

12   Fleishman, Edwin A. *The Structure and Measurement of Physical Fitness.* Englewood Cliffs, NJ: Prentice-Hall, 1964.

13   Clarke, H. Harrison. *Application of Measurement to Health and Physical Education.* Englewood Cliffs, NJ: Prentice-Hall, 1976.

14   Caspersen, Carl J., Kenneth E. Powell, and Gregory M. Christenson. "Physical activity, exercise, and physical fitness: Definitions and distinctions for health-related research." *Public Health Reports* 100, no. 2 (1985): 126-131.

15   American College of Sports Medicine. *ACSM's Guidelines for Exercise Testing and Prescription.* Baltimore, MD: Lippincott Williams & Wilkins, 2006.

16   Pate, Russell R. "The evolving definition of physical fitness." *Quest* 40, no. 3 (1988): 174-179.

17   Penedo, Frank J. and Jason R. Dahn. "Exercise and well-being: A review of mental and physical health benefits associated with physical activity." *Current Opinion in Psychiatry* 18, no. 2 (2005): 189-193.

18   United States Department of Health and Human Services. *Physical Activity and Health: A Report of the Surgeon General.* Atlanta, GA: USDHSS, 1996. Available at https://www.cdc.gov/nccdphp/sgr/pdf/sgrfull.pdf.

19   Rowland, Thomas W. and Patty S. Freedson. "Physical activity, fitness, and health in children: A close look." *Pediatrics* 93, no. 4 (1994): 669-672.

20   Boreham, Colin and Chris Riddoch. "The physical activity, fitness and health of children." *Journal of Sports Sciences* 19, no. 12 (2001): 915-929.

21   Steptoe, Andrew, Jane Wardle, Raymond Fuller, Arne Holte, Joao Justo, Robbert Sanderman, and Lars Wichstrøm. "Leisure-time physical exercise: Prevalence, attitudinal correlates, and behavioral correlates

among young Europeans from 21 countries." *Preventive Medicine* 26, no. 6 (1997): 845-854.

22   Brown, David W., Lina S. Balluz, Gregory W. Heath, David G. Moriarty, Earl S. Ford, Wayne H. Giles, and Ali H. Mokdad. "Associations between recommended levels of physical activity and health-related quality of life: Findings from the 2001 Behavioral Risk Factor Surveillance System (BRFSS) survey." *Preventive Medicine* 37, no. 5 (2003): 520-528.

23   Brown, David W., David R. Brown, Gregory W. Heath, Lina S. Balluz, Wayne H. Giles, Earl S. Ford, and Ali H. Mokdad. "Associations between physical activity dose and health-related quality of life." *Medicine and Science in Sports and Exercise* 36, no. 5 (2004): 890-896.

24   Colcombe, Stanley and Arthur F. Kramer. "Fitness effects on the cognitive function of older adults: A meta-analytic study." *Psychological Science* 14, no. 2 (2003): 125-130.

25   Voss, Michelle W., Timothy B. Weng, Agnieszka Z. Burzynska, Chelsea N. Wong, Gillian E. Cooke, Rachel Clark, Jason Fanning, et al. "Fitness, but not physical activity, is related to functional integrity of brain networks associated with aging." *NeuroImage* 131, no. 1 (2015): 113-115.

26   Larson, Eric B., Li Wang, James D. Bowen, Wayne C. McCormick, Linda Teri, Paul K. Crane, and Walter A Kukull. "Exercise is associated with reduced risk for incident dementia among persons 65 years of age and older." *Annals of Internal Medicine* 144, no. 2 (2006): 73-81.

27   Hammar, Mats and Carl Johan Östgren. "Healthy aging and age-adjusted nutrition and physical fitness." *Best Practice & Research: Clinical Obstetrics & Gynaecology* 27, no. 5 (2013): 741-752.

28   Folkins, Carlyle H. and Wesley E. Sime. "Physical fitness training and mental health." *American Psychologist* 36, no. 4 (1981): 373-389.

29   Plante, Thomas G. and Judith Rodin. "Physical fitness and enhanced psychological health." *Current Psychology* 9, no. 1 (1990): 3-24.

30   Taylor, C. Barr, James F. Sallis, and Richard Needle. "The relation of physical activity and exercise to mental health." *Public Health Reports* 100, no. 2 (1985): 195-202.

31   Paluska, Scott A. and Thomas L. Schwenk. "Physical activity and mental health: Current concepts." *Sports Medicine* 29, no. 3 (2000): 167-180.

32   Diener, Ed. "Subjective well-being: The science of happiness and a proposal for a national index." *American Psychologist* 55, no. 1 (2000): 34-43.

33   Diener, Ed and Martin E.P. Seligman. "Beyond money: Toward an economy of well-being." *Psychological Science in the Public Interest* 5, no. 1 (2004): 1-31.

34   WHOQOL Group. "The World Health Organization quality of life assessment (WHOQOL): Development and general psychometric properties." *Social Science & Medicine* 46, no. 12 (1998): 1569-1585.

35   Galper, Daniel I., Madhukar H. Trivedi, Carolyn E. Barlow, Andrea L. Dunn, and James B. Kampert. "Inverse association between physical inactivity and mental health in men and women." *Medicine and Science in Sports and Exercise* 38, no. 1 (2006): 173-178.

36   Hillman, Charles H., Kirk I. Erickson, and Arthur F. Kramer. "Be smart, exercise your heart: Exercise effects on brain and cognition." *Nature Reviews Neuroscience* 9, no. 1 (2008): 58-65.

37   Bize, Raphaël, Jeffrey A. Johnson, and Ronald C. Plotnikoff. "Physical activity level and health-related quality of life in the general adult population: A systematic review." *Preventive Medicine* 45, no. 6 (2007): 401-415.

38   World Health Organization. *Global Recommendations on Physical Activity for Health*. Geneva: WHO Press, 2010.

39   Vuillemin, Anne, Stéphanie Boini, Sandrine Bertrais, Sabrina Tessier, Jean-Michel Oppert, Serge Hercberg, Francis Guillemin, and Serge Briançon. "Leisure time physical activity and health-related quality of life." *Preventive Medicine* 41, no. 2 (2005): 562-569.

40   Tessier, Sabrina, Anne Vuillemin, Sandrine Bertrais, Stéphanie Boini, Etienne Le Bihan, Jean-Michel Oppert, Serge Hercberg, Francis Guillemin, and Serge Briançon. "Association between leisure-time physical activity and health-related quality of life changes over time." *Preventive Medicine* 44, no. 3 (2007): 202-208.

41   Amarantos, Eleni, Andrea Martinez, and Johanna Dwyer. "Nutrition and quality of life in older adults." *Journals of Gerontology Series A: Biological Sciences and Medical Sciences* 56, suppl. 2 (2001): 54-64.

42   Casey, Patrick H., Kitty L. Szeto, James M. Robbins, Janice E. Stuff, Carol Connell, Jeffery M. Gossett, and Pippa M. Simpson. "Child health-related quality of life and household food security." *Archives of Pediatrics & Adolescent Medicine* 159, no. 1 (2005): 51-56.

43   Keller, Heather H. "Nutrition and health-related quality of life in frail older adults." *Journal of Nutrition, Health & Aging* 8, no. 4 (2003): 245-252.

44   Reedy, Jill, Susan M. Krebs-Smith, Paige E. Miller, Angela D. Liese, Lisa L. Kahle, Yikyung Park, and Amy F. Subar. "Higher diet quality is associated with decreased risk of all-cause, cardiovascular disease, and cancer mortality among older adults." *Journal of Nutrition* 144, no. 6 (2014): 881-889.

45   Guenther, Patricia M., Kellie O. Casavale, Jill Reedy, Sharon I. Kirkpatrick, Hazel AB Hiza, Kevin J. Kuczynski, Lisa L. Kahle, and Susan M. Krebs-Smith. "Update of the healthy eating index: HEI-2010." *Journal of the Academy of Nutrition and Dietetics* 113, no. 4 (2013): 569-580.

46 Bailey, Bruce W., Annette Perkins, Larry A. Tucker, James D. LeCheminant, Jared M. Tucker, and Breckann Moncur. "Adherence to the 2010 dietary guidelines for Americans and the relationship to adiposity in young women." *Journal of Nutrition Education and Behavior* 47, no. 1 (2015): 86-93.

47 Reedy, Jill, Susan M. Krebs-Smith, Paige E. Miller, Angela D. Liese, Lisa L. Kahle, Yikyung Park, and Amy F. Subar. "Higher diet quality is associated with decreased risk of all-cause, cardiovascular disease, and cancer mortality among older adults." *Journal of Nutrition* 144, no. 6 (2014): 881-889.

48 Chiuve, Stephanie E., Teresa T. Fung, Eric B. Rimm, Frank B. Hu, Marjorie L. McCullough, Molin Wang, Meir J. Stampfer, and Walter C. Willett. "Alternative dietary indices both strongly predict risk of chronic disease." *Journal of Nutrition* 142, no. 6 (2012): 1009-1018.

49 Lai, Jun S., Sarah Hiles, Alessandra Bisquera, Alexis J. Hure, Mark McEvoy, and John Attia. "A systematic review and meta-analysis of dietary patterns and depression in community-dwelling adults." *American Journal of Clinical Nutrition* 91, no. 1 (2013): 181-197.

50 Talih, Makram and David T. Huang. "Measuring progress toward target attainment and the elimination of health disparities in healthy people 2020." *Healthy People Statistical Notes*, no. 27 (2016).

51 Penman-Aguilar, Ana, Makram Talih, David Huang, Ramal Moonesinghe, Karen Bouye, and Gloria L. A. Beckles. "Measurement of health disparities, health inequities, and social determinants of health to support the advancement of health equity." *Journal of Public Health Management and Practice* 22, suppl. 1 (2016): S33-42.

52 World Health Organization (WHO). "The seven dimensions of wellness." (2007).

53 Hoeger, Wener W. K. and Sharon A. Hoeger. *Lifetime Physical Fitness and Wellness: A Personalized Program*. Stamford, CT: Cengage Learning, 2016.

54 World Health Organization (WHO). "The seven dimensions of wellness." (2007).

55 Office of Disease Prevention and Health Promotion. "2008 Physical Activity Guidelines for Americans Summary." http://health.gov/paguidelines/guidelines/summary.aspx.

56 Centers for Disease Control and Prevention. "Steps to Wellness: A Guide to Implementing the 2008 Physical Activity Guidelines for Americans." Atlanta: US Department of Health and Human Services, 2012.

57 Singh, Anita, Tamara L. Bennett, and Patricia A. Deuster. *Force Health Protection: Nutrition and Exercise Resource Manual*. Department of Military and Emergency Medicine Uniformed Services University of the Health Sciences, 1999, 29.

58 Centers for Disease Control and Prevention. "Steps to Wellness: A Guide to Implementing the 2008 Physical Activity Guidelines for Americans." Atlanta: US Department of Health and Human Services, 2012.

59 Ainsworth, B. E., W. L. Haskell, S. D. Herrmann, N. Meckes, D. R. Bassett, C. Tudor- Locke, J. L. Greer, J. Vezina, M. C. Whitt-Glover, and A. S. Leon. "The Compendium of Physical Activities Tracking Guide." Healthy Lifestyles Research Center, College of Nursing & Health Innovation, Arizona State University." https://sites.google.com/site/compendiumofphysicalactivities.

60 Humphrey, Reed. "Clinical applications: The exercise caloric challenge." *ACSM's Health & Fitness Journal* 10, no. 2 (2006): 40-41.

61 Bushman, Barbara A. "Wouldn't you like to know: How can I use METs to quantify the amount of aerobic exercise?" *ACSM's Health & Fitness Journal* 16, no. 2 (2012): 5-7.

62 Nes, Bjarne M., Imre Janszky, Lars J. Vatten, Tom I. Nilsen, Stian T. Aspenes, and Ulrick Wisløff. "Estimating VO$_2$ peak from a nonexercise prediction model: The HUNT study, Norway." *Medicine & Science in Sports & Exercise* 43, no. 11 (2011): 2024-2030.

63 Norwegian University of Science and Technology. "Fitness Calculator." http://www.ntnu.edu/cerg/vo2max.

64 Reedy, Jill, Susan M. Krebs-Smith, Paige E. Miller, Angela D. Liese, Lisa L. Kahle, Yikyung Park, and Amy F. Subar. "Higher diet quality is associated with decreased risk of all-cause, cardiovascular disease, and cancer mortality among older adults." *Journal of Nutrition* 144, no. 6 (2014): 881-889.

65 US Department of Health and Human Services and US Department of Agriculture. *2015–2020 Dietary Guidelines for Americans*, 8th ed. December 2015. http://health.gov/dietaryguidelines/2015/guidelines/.

66 DeSalvo, Karen B., Richard Olson, and Kellie O. Casavale. "Dietary guidelines for Americans." *Journal of the American Medical Association* 315, no. 5 (2016): 457-458.

67 World Health Organization (WHO). *Health 2020. A European Policy Framework and Strategy for the 21st Century*. Copenhagen: WHO, 2015.

68 US Department of Agriculture. "My Plate, My State: Washington, DC." www.choosemyplate.gov.

69 US Department of Agriculture. "Supertracker: Sample Meal Plans." https:// supertracker.usda.gov/samplemealplans.aspx.

70 Epel, Elissa, Sherlyn Jimenez, Kelly Brownell, Laura R. Stroud, Catherine M. Stoney, and Ray Niaura. "Are stress eaters at risk for the metabolic syndrome?" *Annals of the New York Academy of Sciences* 1032, no. 1 (2005): 208-210.

71 Torres, Susan J. and Caryl A. Nowson. "Relationship between stress, eating behavior, and obesity," *Nutrition* 23, no. 11-12 (2007): 887-894.

72   Kivimäki, Mika, Jenny A. Head, Jane E. Ferrie, Martin J. Shipley, Eric J. Brunner, Jussi Vahtera, and Michael Marmot. "Work stress, weight gain and weight loss: Evidence for bidirectional effects of job strain on body mass index in the Whitehall II study." *International Journal of Obesity* 30, no. 6 (2006): 982-987.

73   Räikkönen, Katri, Karen A. Matthews, and Lewis H. Kuller. "Depressive symptoms and stressful life events predict metabolic syndrome among middle-aged women: A comparison of World Health Organization, Adult Treatment Panel III, and International Diabetes Foundation definitions." *Diabetes Care* 30, no. 4 (2007): 872-877.

74   Ford, Earl S., Wayne H. Giles, and Ali H. Mokdad. "Increasing prevalence of the metabolic syndrome among US adults." *Diabetes Care* 27, no. 10 (2004): 2444-2449.

75   Marchesini, Giulio, Elisabetta Bugianesi, Gabriele Forlani, Fernanda Cerrelli, Marco Lenzi, Rita Manini, Stefania Natale, et al. "Nonalcoholic fatty liver, steatohepatitis, and the metabolic syndrome." *Hepatology* 37, no. 4 (2003): 917-923.

76   Esposito, Katherine, Paolo Chiodini, Annamaria Colao, Andrea Lenzi, and Dario Giugliano. "Metabolic syndrome and risk of cancer: A systematic review and meta-analysis." *Diabetes Care* 35, no. 11 (2012): 2402-241.

77   Pearson, Erin S. "Goal setting as a health behavior change strategy in overweight and obese adults: A systematic literature review examining intervention components." *Patient Education and Counseling* 87, no. 1 (2012): 32-42.

78   Willett, Walter C. *Eat, Drink, and Be Healthy: The Harvard Medical School Guide to Healthy Eating.* New York: Simon and Schuster, 2001.

79   Goff, David C., Donald M. Lloyd-Jones, Glen Bennett, Sean Coady, Ralph B. D'Agostino, Raymond Gibbons, Philip Greenland, et al. "2013 ACC/AHA guideline on the assessment of cardiovascular risk: A report of the American College of Cardiology/American Heart Association Task Force on Practice Guidelines." *Circulation* 129, no. 25, suppl. 2 (2014): S49-73.

80   Preedy, Victor R., Lan-Anh Hunter, and Vinood B. Patel, eds. *Diet Quality: An Evidence-Based Approach* vol. 2. New York: Humana Press, 2013.

81   Mitrou, Panagiota N., Victor Kipnis, Anne C M Thiébaut, Jill Reedy, Amy F. Subar, Elisabet Wirfält, Andrew Flood, et al. "Mediterranean dietary pattern and prediction of all-cause mortality in a US population: Results from the NIH-AARP Diet and Health Study." *Archives of Internal Medicine* 167, no. 22 (2008): 2461-2468.

82   Fung, Teresa T., Kathryn M. Rexrode, Christos S. Mantzoros, JoAnn E. Manson, Walter C. Willett, and Frank B. Hu. "Mediterranean diet and incidence of and mortality from coronary heart disease and stroke in women." *Circulation* 119, no. 8 (2009): 1093-1100.

83   Trichopoulou, Antonia, Philippos Orfanos, Teresa Norat, Bas Bueno-de-Mesquita, Marga C. Ocké, Petra HM Peeters, Yvonne T. van der Schouw, et al. "Modified Mediterranean diet and survival: EPIC-elderly prospective cohort study." *BMJ* 330, no. 7498 (2005): 991.

84   Fung, Teresa T., Stephanie E. Chiuve, Marjorie L. McCullough, Kathryn M. Rexrode, Giancarlo Logroscino, and Frank B. Hu. "Adherence to a DASH-style diet and risk of coronary heart disease and stroke in women." *Archives of Internal Medicine* 168, no. 7 (2008): 713-720.

85   US Dept. of Health & Human Services, National Heart, Lung, and Blood Institute. "Description of the DASH Eating Plan." https://www.nhlbi.nih.gov/health-topics/dash-eating-plan.

86   Mayo Clinic. "Sample menus for the DASH diet." https://www.mayoclinic.org/healthy-lifestyle/nutrition-and-healthy-eating/in-depth/dash-diet/art-20047110.

87   National Institutes of Health. "Following the DASH Eating Plan." NIH Publication No. 06-5834. https://www.nhlbi.nih.gov/files/docs/public/heart/dash_brief.pdf.

88   Sacks, Frank M., Laura P. Svetkey, William M. Vollmer, Lawrence J. Appel, George A. Bray, David Harsha, Eva Obarzanek, et al. "Effects on blood pressure of reduced dietary sodium and the Dietary Approaches to Stop Hypertension (DASH) diet." *New England Journal of Medicine* 344, no. 1 (2001): 3-10.

89   Vollmer, William M., Frank M. Sacks, Jamy Ard, Lawrence J. Appel, George A. Bray, Denise G. Simons-Morton, Paul R. Conlin, et al. "Effects of diet and sodium intake on blood pressure: Subgroup analysis of the DASH-sodium trial." *Annals of Internal Medicine* 135, no. 12 (2001): 1019-1028.

90   Blumenthal, James A., Michael A. Babyak, Alan Hinderliter, Lana L. Watkins, Linda Craighead, Pao-Hwa Lin, Carla Caccia, Julie Johnson, Robert Waugh, and Andrew Sherwood. "Effects of the DASH diet alone and in combination with exercise and weight loss on blood pressure and cardiovascular biomarkers in men and women with high blood pressure: The ENCORE study." *Archives of Internal Medicine* 170, no. 2 (2010): 126-135.

91   Appel, Lawrence J., Catherine M. Champagne, David W. Harsha, Lawton S. Cooper, Eva Obarzanek, Patricia J. Elmer, Victor J. Stevens, et al. "Effects of comprehensive lifestyle modification on blood pressure control: Main results of the PREMIER clinical trial." *Journal of the American Medical Association* 289, no. 16 (2003): 2083-2093.

92   Soltani, Sepideh, Fatemeh Shirani, Maryam J. Chitsazi, and Amin Salehi-Abargouei. "The effect of dietary approaches to stop hypertension (DASH) diet on weight and body composition in adults: A systematic review and meta-analysis of randomized controlled clinical trials." *Obesity Reviews* 17, no. 5 (2016): 442-454.

93   Kristjánsson, Álfgeir Logi, Inga Dóra Sigfúsdóttir, and John P. Allegrante. "Health behavior and academic

achievement among adolescents: The relative contribution of dietary habits, physical activity, body mass index, and self-esteem." *Health Education & Behavior* 37, no. 1 (2010): 51-64.

94   Office of Disease Prevention and Health Promotion. "Healthy People 2020." http://www.healthypeople.gov/2020/default.aspx.

95   National Association for Sport and Physical Education/American Heart Association. "2012 Shape of the Nation Report: Status of Physical Education in the USA." http://www.shapeamerica.org/advocacy/son/2012/upload/2012-Shape-of-Nation-full-report-web.pdf.

96   Schilling, Joseph and Jonathan Logan. "Greening the rust belt: A green infrastructure model for right sizing America's shrinking cities." *Journal of the American Planning Association* 74, no. 4 (2008): 451-466.

97   Lopez, Steve. *Reorganizing the Rust Belt: An Inside Study of the American Labor Movement.* Berkeley and Los Angeles: University of California Press, 2004.

3

RELAXATION

Sometimes the most important thing in a whole day
is the rest we take between two deep breaths.

— Etty Hillesum

OVERVIEW

Why: Relax to reduce the reaction to stress and break the cycle of arousal, hypervigilance, and escalating stress. Relaxation reduces tension and stress through processes that lower metabolic rate. Practice relaxation as an aid for getting to sleep (fig 3–1).

How: Obtain a baseline level of stress, perform a *relaxation* exercise, and remeasure the level of stress.

Identifying a measure of change between before and then after developing the goal and steps to meet the goal provides us a measure of our success. We use the Subjective Units of Distress Scale (SUDS) to help subjectively identify the stress level before, and again after, as somewhere between zero (0) and ten (10), where 0 corresponds to no stress and 10 to the highest level of stress you have ever experienced. The anticipation is that the SUDS level begins to decrease even after developing a goal statement and the steps to attain the goal. If the SUDS level increases, then take some time to reassess the goal statement to assure it is attainable. And reassess the steps to assure that they have been adequately defined and there are a sufficient number. After all, you want to be able to check off each step and mark progress toward reaching your goal.

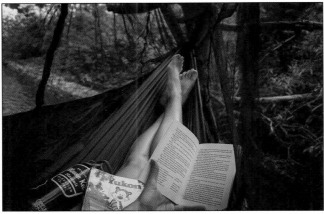

Fig. 3–1. Relaxation reduces tension and stress. (unsplash.com)

Goal Setting Skill—Relaxation

Have you ever stopped to think about how to relax? If so, how do you relax? If not, let's explore together.

Rate the stress level you perceive

Analog SUDS	Digital SUDS	Emoji SUDS
Actually, I'm not stressed	0	
A little stressed	1–3	
Somewhat stressed	4–6	
Quite a bit stressed	7–8	
It's really bad	9	
Run and hide!!	10	

Think about what's stressing you out. What might help?

Try and identify an objective to help you do that.

Now it's time to figure out how to get there.

Write out your relaxation goal statement and how you plan to get there, step-by-step.

Use the systems below as suggested approaches.

Now get started! Don't be shy. Go for it!

Have you made any progress?

Rate the stress level you perceive now

Is it lower?

Yes	No
Congratulations!! You did it!! Now you can do this whenever you need it!	What might have gone wrong? Did you figure out all your steps? Did you actually do them all? Did you give yourself enough time? Give it another try, from the beginning.

Is SUDS the only option for measuring change? Certainly not! You are encouraged to find the most appropriate measurement for your needs. The only thing that matters is that it can provide meaningful feedback with regard to change, or even transformation, resulting from applying the goal-setting process. Perhaps a scale that measures the likelihood of completing the task might be more useful. That scale might range from 0 to 10, where 0 corresponds to zero chance of completion and 10 is fully sure of completion. If you were using a likelihood-of-completion scale, then you would anticipate an increase in likelihood to complete from premeasure to postmeasure.

The listings and descriptions below are representative of the most thoroughly documented and commonly used relaxation approaches. Take a look and see which one(s) seems most attractive to you. Try each of your choices in the SUDS framework and work further with the one that proves to be the best fit.

- Diaphragmatic breathing, or *eupnoea*, is slow breathing with your focus concentrating on the movement of your diaphragm. Focus, too, on the word *relax* each time you exhale.

- Alternate nostril breathing is similar to diaphragmatic breathing but uses the thumb and index finger to close one nostril to inhale, switching and closing the other nostril to exhale.

- Progressive muscle relaxation (PMR) helps to bring awareness of your body by focusing on slowly tensing and then relaxing each muscle group in sequence.[1,2]

- Positive imagery, or *visualization*, is the forming of mental images of a peaceful, calm place or situation. The idea is to get lost in the image by using your sight, smell, hearing, and touch.

- Social resilience model (SRM) uses stabilization skills to reduce and prevent the symptoms of stress. In its simplest form, SRM focuses on accessing the parasympathetic system through several processes.[3]

- Mindfulness-based stress reduction (MBSR) is the practice of bringing awareness to the present moment.[4,5,6]

- Good sleep hygiene is accomplished by maintaining a consistent sleep-wake schedule, exercising daily, minimizing caffeine and alcohol consumption as bedtime nears, and eliminating long naps and naps within a few hours of bedtime.

WHY RELAXATION?

It's not that all stress is bad. In fact, our survival as individuals, as a tribe, and as a species has been dependent on our adaptation to stress. Without a certain amount of stress, we will not grow. Welcoming stress that can engage the sympathetic part of our autonomic nervous system can be a good thing, especially if we are in situations that demand our full and immediate attention. An ER nurse responding to a code blue is activating the sympathetic nervous system, as is the first responder heading for a mass casualty incident or a firefighter running into a burning building. That this is happening to us in those stressful moments can be a good thing. In some cases, it can save our lives. During training sessions, we often explain this by relating it to emergency medical technicians who approach a victim of an auto accident. We don't want the EMTs mellow and relaxed, nor do we want them paralyzed with terror. We want them in control of themselves and the situation. And I am sure those of you in the first responder community want that for yourselves as well.

Think of your autonomic nervous system as a car alarm (fig. 3–2). When there is danger or threat, the alarm goes off; when the threat is gone, the alarm turns off. Robert Sapolsky observed in his book *Why Zebras Don't Get Ulcers* that, in the animal kingdom, stress is episodic and once the threat is gone, animals will return to homeostasis or balance.[7] As we humans have evolved and become more civilized, our stress is no longer episodic but chronic. In other words, the car alarm will now go off when a butterfly lands on the windshield. While this may be a funny image, the physical and psychological consequences to us, especially in the caregiving community, is not humorous.[8,9,10,11] Consider that cardio-respiratory and gastrointestinal problems are significantly higher among those with PTSD.[12] Epidemiologic research increasingly suggests that exposure to traumatic events is associated with increased health care utilization, negative health outcomes, the onset of specific diseases, and even early death. Clinical studies have confirmed the prevalence of common autoimmune diseases, including rheumatoid arthritis, psoriasis, insulin-dependent diabetes, and thyroid disease, to such chronic stresses.[13] The crucial point here is that problems arise when we can't access the parasympathetic portion of our autonomic nervous system.

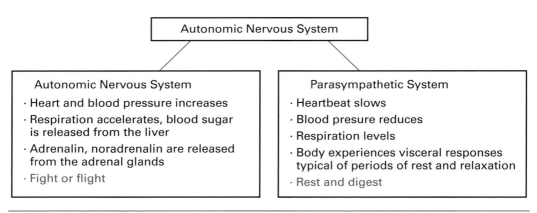

Fig. 3–2. The autonomic nervous system acts largely unconsciously.

We all have incredibly busy and demanding lives, and while the 2015 "Stress in America" survey completed by the American Psychological Association showed a slight drop in stress levels overall, it also revealed that nearly 25% of the some 3,000 people surveyed reported experiencing extreme stress, compared to 18% in 2014.[14] As a side note, Americans have approximately half the vacation time as Europeans.[15] Compounding this is the fact that an estimated 50–70 million U.S. adults have sleep and/or wakefulness disorders.[16] In the caring professions, these two factors lead to increased errors, poor quality of life, increased health problems, and even early death. Yes, poor sleep quality can actually kill us. For example, it is estimated that first responders will live, on average, 15 years less than the general population.[17] One of the major factors is poor sleep due to shift work, sleep disruption, nightmares, and poor sleep quality.[18,19,20] The impact of poor sleep can impact student performance, medical decision making, and caregiver long-term health.[21,22,23,24]

THE HOW OF RELAXATION

Breathing is the most basic life-giving thing we do, yet we seldom pay attention to how we breathe (fig. 3–3). In times of stress, breathing tends to get rapid and shallow because the body is on alert. These changes in breathing patterns arise from the body's potential need for more oxygen than usual to either escape or fight. By learning to pay attention and changing our breathing, we can reduce our reaction to stress. This, in turn, helps to break the cycle of arousal, hypervigilance, and escalating stress.

The human body constantly gives off cues that it is stressed, but what happens over time if we ignore those internal messages? That's right, there is a huge physical and mental toll, as illustrated above. So, in this chapter, we focus on paying attention to those cues, learning to breathe correctly, and activating our relaxation response. This can help us with our sleep as well.

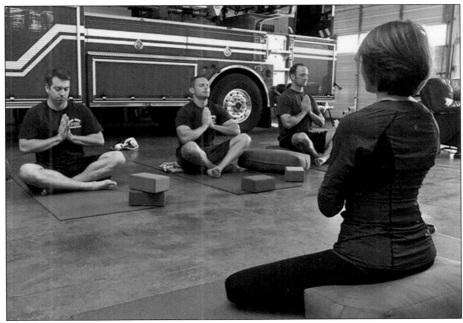

Fig. 3–3. Firefighters who practice yoga learn how to breathe. (Courtesy of FlexYoga.)

There are multitudes of ways we can relax. The simple act of listening to music can reduce stress.[25] And don't forget about pets and hobbies!

Consider using a relaxation practice log (fig. 3–4). Note the date of the activity, your initial SUDS level, the focal point of the physical stress you are feeling, the relaxation skill you used, the length of time you used the relaxation skill, and your subsequent SUDS level. While it may seem silly and some may resist the idea of keeping a log, research has clearly demonstrated that these devices can increase our likelihood of success in changing attitude and behavior.[26,27,28]

RELAXATION PRACTICE LOG					
Date	**SUDS (0–10)**	**Where do you feel stress in your body?**	**Skill Practiced**	**Minutes**	**SUDS (0–10)**

Fig. 3–4. Sample relaxation worksheet

Case Study: A student is anticipating an important mid-term exam. The student decides to do a relaxation exercise. As a group discussion and to familiarize ourselves with the relaxation practice log worksheet, how might we develop the student's relaxation worksheet?

RELAXATION PRACTICE LOG

Date	SUDS (0–10)	Where do you feel stress in your body?	Skill Practiced	Minutes	SUDS (0–10)
2/24/18	4	Upper back	Diaphragmatic breathing	10	1

Reflect: What is your SUDS score right now? (0–10) _____

Diaphragmatic breathing

Diaphragmatic breathing is a breathing-related relaxation skill that is easy to master.[29,30] The thoracic diaphragm, the sheet of muscle just below our rib cage, serves as the primary muscle mechanism for breathing. While all of us use our diaphragmatic muscle when breathing, few of us are consciously aware of its activity, and even fewer of us focus on developing the diaphragm through breathing exercises.

When using your diaphragm to its greatest advantage, the area of the abdomen directly beneath the rib cage flexes visibly, drawing air into the lungs efficiently. This is in contrast to inefficient shallow breathing, in which the muscles around the rib cage flex more prominently. Infants and young children deeply flex their diaphragms when breathing, while many adults visibly flex the muscles around the chest. While flexing the rib cage may cut a more imposing figure, it might not always be the most beneficial way to breathe.

Simple breathing exercises can help us focus on diaphragmatic breathing and the development of this essential muscle. To practice diaphragmatic breathing, simply get comfortable in your chair or lie on the floor and put one hand on your chest and the other on your upper abdomen. As you breathe, do so slowly and focus on encouraging your abdominal cavity to expand, subsequently causing the hand on your abdomen to move upward. The movement of your rib cage should be minimal and the hand on your chest should remain relatively still. As you exhale, focus on the word *relax*. Do this breathing exercise for 2 minutes. Diaphragmatic breathing is a practical example of classical conditioning or associative learning, where two unrelated things become associated in a person's mind. When practicing diaphragmatic breathing, focusing on the word *relax* becomes associated with the process of relaxation and, over time, the word itself can become a trigger for the process of relaxation.

Reflect: What has your SUDS level become now and what changes do notice in your body?

_____

_____

_____

_____

Alternate nostril breathing

Alternate nostril breathing is yet another breathing-related relaxation skill.[31] This is a yogic breathing technique wherein the practitioner inhales through one nostril and exhales through the other. To practice alternate nostril breathing, take your thumb and index finger and place your thumb on one nostril, closing it. Next, breathe in through the open nostril. When you have taken in a full breath, release your thumb from the nostril. Close the other nostril with your index finger and exhale. Do this slowly five times. Reverse the process, closing the opposite nostril with your index finger and inhaling, then closing the remaining nostril with your thumb and exhaling. As you exhale, focus on the word *relax*. Do this slowly, also five times.

Reflect: What has your SUDS level become now and what changes do notice in your body?

_____

_____

_____

_____

Progressive muscle relaxation

Progressive muscle relaxation (PMR) is another relaxation technique. This one is different, though, in that it can help encourage awareness of the body.[32,33] PMR is a skill that can be used in a variety of situations to promote relaxation. During the PMR training process, the practitioner moves through the entire body sequentially, tensing and relaxing all of the major muscle groups, one group at a time. Please, please don't think you have to tense any injured areas of the body.

This process begins as with the earlier relaxation activities: with a focus on breathing. Practice diaphragmatic breathing, inhaling and exhaling. Allow yourself to close your eyes as you focus on your breathing. With each exhale imagine yourself saying the word *relax*. Now, start with your feet and work your way up to the top of your head. Tense your feet, then focus on the word *relax* and let go of the tension in your feet. Do the same for your calf muscles, then the muscles in your thighs. Continue this process with every muscle group until you reach the muscles in your forehead, always focusing on the word *relax* when letting go of the tension.

Once you have gone through your entire body using the PMR technique, imagine yourself in a relaxing, calm place. For example, this place might be on an island, on a beach, or in the mountains by a lake or a stream. This exercise will probably require about 15 minutes. Please give it the time it deserves.

Reflect: What has your SUDS level become now and what changes do you notice in your body?

_____

_____

_____

_____

Social resilience model

The social resilience model (SRM) uses stabilization skills to reduce and prevent the symptoms of stress. In its simplest form, SRM focuses on accessing the parasympathetic system through any of several processes.

- Grounding is a technique where we focus our attention on physical contact with a stable surface. It may be accomplished while sitting, standing, or lying down with the goal of establishing a sense of self and foundational safety. The process is intended to focus attention on the present moment by finding a comfortable body position and noticing, or bringing our attention to, how your body is being supported and the associated physical sensations. Like most skills, this needs to be practiced, but requires less time as it becomes more familiar.[34]

- Resourcing is a way to focus on positive or neutral factors to build sensations of regulation. It uses either external resources, such as positive experiences or memories of people, places, or activities, or internal resources, such as values, beliefs, or positive personal characteristics. The intent is to identify your resources and experience the sensations associated with the resource. This process stabilizes the nervous system and promotes well-being and embodiment. For those having difficulty with grounding or who find the experience unpleasant, resourcing may be attractive.

- Resource intensification is used by expanding our attention to the multisensory details of the resource. This skill is intended to expand the time spent with the resource by considering the all of the sensory aspects of the resource, such as sounds, smells, tastes, and images. This process builds self-regulation and brings awareness to the notion that sensations can be uncomfortable, neutral, or positive.

Mindfulness-based stress reduction

Mindfulness-based stress reduction (MBSR) is the practice of awareness in the present moment.[35,36] While this may seem like an easy task, it can be harder than one thinks. For most of us, our minds can wander to future-land, where we create worries and stress for ourselves with thoughts of what we should or shouldn't do. If our minds get bored with projecting into the future, we can always journey to past-land, where we can exhume old regrets and memories that result in guilt and shame. Neither of these terrains offer us less stress. In the practice of MSBR, one learns to be in the here-and-now physically, mentally, and spiritually.[37,38,39,40]

Most of us believe that we are pretty mindful, but a colleague who does resiliency training uses the raisin exercise to illustrate how difficult being focused and mindful can be.[41] This exercise is designed to teach students just how hard staying focused can be.

Give each student a small box of raisins and explain the following rules for the exercise:

1. When the instructed to do so, each student places one raisin in their mouth.

2. They will keep the raisin in their mouth for 90 seconds. Important note: No one is allowed to keep time other than the instructor.

3. They are not to chew or swallow the raisin, nor are they allowed to park it in a corner of their mouth. Instead they will need to continually move the raisin around, concentrating on the raisin's texture, taste, and where it currently is in their mouth. They must have some remnant of the raisin remaining in their mouth at the end of the 90-second exercise.

4. Most importantly, it is critical that each student's only focus is on the raisin. Each time their mind begins to drift ("gosh, this is a stupid exercise" or "I have to get ready for tomorrow's meeting") they must refocus on the raisin, once again becoming aware of its texture, flavor, and so on.

The exercise is also designed to activate the executive control network of the brain, whose function is to cause us to focus on the moment—being present. Interestingly, research has shown that practicing mindfulness for just eight weeks can bring about positive changes in the gray matter of the brain, providing cognitive and psychological benefits lasting through-out the day.[42]

After the exercise, ask each participant how long he or she believes the exercise lasted. Although armed with the knowledge beforehand that the exercise lasts for only 90 seconds, many students will feel it seemed like an eternity, while others perceive the exercise was over in the blink of an eye.

Reflect: No matter which skill you use, notice changes in your SUDS level after practicing the skill. What changes do you notice in your body?

_____

_____

_____

_____

Practice makes perfect. Consider the following:

- Create a Relaxation Practice Log.
- Keep a daily SUDS log until your SUDS level is reduced to a 2 with some consistency.
- Practice a relaxation exercise two to four times a day.

> *One way to break up any kind of tension is good deep breathing.*
> — Byron Nelson

INTERNALIZE RELAXATION

Think of a time in your life when you were stressed about something and you were able to take a couple of deep breaths and get yourself calmed down. Think about where you were, what you were thinking, and what physical sensations you had while you thought about this situation (fig. 3–5). What changed as you took those deep breaths? Did your heart rate and breathing slow down? What was your SUDS level during that time of stress before you took those few breaths and what was it afterward?

Precalming SUDS: _____

Postcalming SUDS: _____

As you think back on that event, how confident do you feel going forward that you can use a relaxation skill as a tool to help you cope with the stress you will confront?

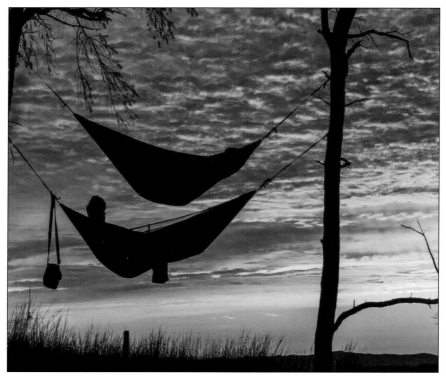

Fig. 3–5. Think about a time when you were stressed and how you calmed yourself down. (unsplash.com)

EXTERNALIZE: APPLY RELAXATION AS A GROUP

We've looked at several relaxation exercises, including diaphragmatic breathing, alternate nostril breathing, progressive muscle relaxation, mindfulness-based stress reduction, and the social resilience model. Given these tools, examine the following case study.

Case study: You and your friend are involved in a relatively minor car crash incident and there are no apparent injuries. Your friend, the driver, is visibly agitated and breathing rapidly. After a thorough physical assessment by a paramedic, it is determined there are no injuries and all vital signs are within normal limits. And, after contacting medical control, the decision is that both drivers are competent to refuse further treatment. Your friend is upset because of the damage to the new vehicle and is afraid it will cause the auto insurance premium to increase. Your friend is having some difficulty attempting to calm down at this time. How would you react to this situation and what intervention would you provide?

> *I might add that it would be best not to tell your friend to "calm down." If the friend is like me, and probably like most of us, telling the friend to calm down will only increase their irritation and stress reaction. In these and similar situations, it is best to model what we are suggesting to the other person. If we slow down our own breathing and model that, we increase the likelihood they will begin to synchronize their breathing with ours.[42] Also remember that you can use any of the other skills we've discussed. So, for example, if your friend is really stressed, it may be best to get him or her moving around to dissipate some of the stress hormones. In that way, physical activity would be useful here.*

Reflect: Using think-aloud pair problem solving (TAPPS), collaborative groups will develop a possible intervention to the case study.

Identify prerelaxation exercise SUDS (0–10), relaxation method, and post-relaxation exercise SUDS (0–10).

Prerelaxation SUDS (0–10): _____

Relaxation method: _____

Postrelaxation SUDS (0–10): _____

PRACTICE RELAXATION

Observe, record, tabulate, communicate. Use your five senses.
Learn to see, learn to hear, learn to feel, learn to smell,
and know that by practice alone you can become expert.

— William Olser, MD

To become an expert of any skill we have to practice it and this is true for learning to relax (fig. 3–6). Yes, it is a sad commentary about our culture that we actually have to practice how to relax.

Remember, resilient people do not live in a pie-in-the-sky world. They understand that they need to train for the times when their resilience skills will be needed. Another way to think of this is if you noticed a decrease in your SUDS using the diaphragmatic breathing skill, wouldn't you be worth a total of 8 minutes a day to refine this lifesaving skill? Too often we've seen people who will learn a relaxation skill and then try to use it only when they are really stressed. In their disappointment, they will complain that it didn't work. And they are right, but not because the skill didn't work. It's because they didn't refine the skill or make it a habit in their lives. Incorporating any relaxation skill—whether it be yoga, Tai chi, meditation, or the skills we've discussion here—into our daily lives can have a positive impact on our physical and mental health. As I mentioned in the goal-setting module, the self-discipline of creating a practice or habit increases our self-confidence and our belief in ourselves. So, consider one of the relaxation skills you can use today to cope with the stresses in your life.

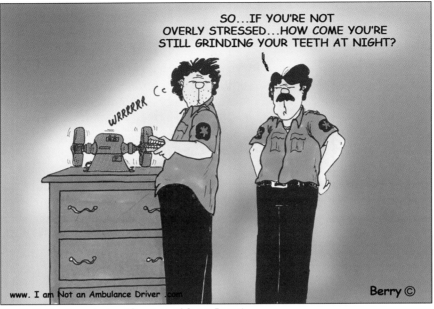

Fig. 3–6. Practice relaxing. (Courtesy of Steve Berry.)

Activity: Create a specific plan for practicing an exercise with the goal of being sufficiently practiced so that you need only briefly meditate on your relaxation word to bring about the desired results.

Reflect: Does developing a relaxation plan and practicing the plan over several weeks make a difference in your ability to relax after a stressful encounter? Why?

_____

_____

_____

_____

The difference between ordinary and extraordinary is practice.

— Vladimir Horowitz

APPLY RELAXATION TO YOUR COMMUNITY

I once had a young boy with severe asthma as a patient who was able to reduce the number of attacks and their intensity by becoming skilled at controlling his breathing.[43,44,45] In fact, he got so good at it he began to teach diaphragmatic breathing to

> *his whole family. He reported that they would gather in the living room, lie on the floor, and listen to a relaxation tape I had made for him. The entire family learned to be less reactive to his asthma attacks, which helped him, and they created a positive chain rather than becoming caught in a vicious cycle of fear and stress.*[46]

This is an example of how you can apply these techniques to your community. A community can be a team, department, family, neighborhood, town, and so on. Establishing and maintaining a good support system is essential to effective resiliency as a source of strength and as an opportunity to offer support to others. Teaching and modeling relaxation skills to those in our support system is an easy way that we can be mentors to those we care about.

Activity: What are the implications of expanding this skill to a community, where community is defined as any group of people living and/or working together in one place?

Think about the following discussion points:

- Define the community where you are intending to apply the skill.
- Identify why this skill is appropriate for the particular community.
- Consider how the skill would be administered and sustained.

Reflect: How important is it to your community to be able to establish a relaxation skills program? If you are a first responder, does establishing a relaxation plan at a community level decrease the immediate stress after a difficult incident? If you are a student, does teaching relaxation skills to your study group or study partner increase your confidence going into an important exam, while decreasing your stress? [47,48]

SLEEP

Without enough sleep, we all become tall two-year-olds.

— JoJo Jensen

Why: Some 40% of Americans sleep 5 hours or less each night. Without adequate sleep we are twice as likely to suffer from heart disease and 1.7 times more likely to die from all other diseases.[49] One of the great myths about sleep hygiene is "I can take control of my sleep if I focus on increasing the number of hours of sleep I get." Rather, it is the quality of sleep that gives us restful, refreshing sleep. Sleep problems are rooted in the quality of sleep, not the quantity of sleep. We have all had sleepless nights, only to arise in the morning to guzzle coffee and stuff ourselves with sugary foods, hoping to boost our energy and clear our minds. While this may be a temporary solution, we all know how we feel a few hours later, and most certainly by the afternoon we are neither performing at our best nor are we able to handle stressful situations in a resilient way. We are typically more irritable, our listening skills are diminished, and our problem-solving abilities are impaired. Without quality sleep our performance and judgment are dramatically compromised.[50,51] And those who have to do shift work are at greater risk for physical and psychological problems.[52,53] For college students, poor sleep hygiene can have a significant impact on academic performance.[54,55] Physiological impairments can include heart rate variability, decreased reaction time, tremors, aches, weakened immune system, decreased body temperature, and increased risks such as heart disease, diabetes, obesity, and growth suppression.

Disrupted sleep patterns are a recognized source of stress for emergency service workers. In one study of over 700 firefighters, one-third reported sleep disturbances (disruption, poor-quality sleep, not enough sleep) as a critical cause of stress.[56] The relationship between sleep deprivation and decreased performance is well documented. For example, being awake for 18 hours produces degeneration equal to a blood alcohol content of 0.05%,[57] which in many countries means we're legally drunk. A lack of sleep has been shown to negatively impact learning capacity and academic performance.[58,59,60] For example, efforts by students to pull all-nighters to cram for tests may result in depression and even poorer academic performance.[61]

Attempts to use alcohol to get to sleep only compound the problem as it decreases what is known as stage IV or dream sleep, also known as rapid eye movement (REM) sleep.[62,63] This phenomenon can be followed by an increase in REM activity as the night progresses. So, while alcohol will decrease REM activity early in the sleep cycles, there can be increases in REM activity at the end of the night that cause multiple awakenings and, for some individuals, can increase the recall of nightmares and vivid dreams. Further, even young healthy males can show a decrease in personal performance and an increase in anxiety upon waking after using alcohol to sleep.[64]

Individuals with post-traumatic stress disorder (PTSD) show worsened sleep problems because of persistent nightmares and hyperarousal. These symptoms increase the likelihood of individuals trying to avoid sleep and creating a problematic sleep cycle. Why? Because when sleep finally occurs, the brain tries to make up for deprivation of the REM sleep stage.

A general understanding of how we sleep can help us understand how sleep affects our performance. Sleep is a somewhat sequential process whereby we go through five to six cycles of staged sleep lasting about 90 minutes.[65] These stages of sleep can be linked to bodily functions. The first stage of sleep lasts up to 15 minutes and helps us transition to deeper second-stage sleep. The second stage of sleep, lasting about 20 minutes, addresses muscle relaxation and possibly memory consolidation. Awakening at this stage would bring about a sense of alertness, making this ideal for naps. The third stage is associated with slower brain wave activity and has been linked to restorative bodily functions such as muscle repair. Awakening at this stage would find one feeling groggy and irritable. The third stage lasts about 60 minutes, but becomes shorter in length as the sleep cycles are repeated. Stage IV sleep is when most of the dreaming appears to occur.

How: We cannot truly control our sleep. In fact, the more we try to control sleep the more likely we are to stay awake. Sleep is about letting go and simply letting sleep happen. There are actions that can help to facilitate sleep, however. If you can't get to sleep within 15–20 minutes, get out of bed and consider some nonstressful activity until you become sleepy. When you are sleepy, return to bed. Repeat if necessary as you are establishing a behavior.

The following tips are also recommended for those who have trouble getting to sleep. Make a purposeful effort to slow down 20 to 60 minutes before bed. Avoid caffeine, cigarette smoking, or alcohol. Sleep in a cool and dark room, and adults should limit activities in bed to sleep and sex. Avoid looking at your clock when you wake up in the night. Practice positive imagery. Take time to reflect on what you are grateful for. When possible, get up at the same time every day. Avoid naps, especially in the late afternoon, and limit them to 45 minutes. Make your bed each morning. This simple activity will reward you. Use image rehearsal training, which is a process to change a nightmare into a more controlled dream.

Create a sleep log to aid in identifying your sleep patterns (fig. 3–7). Sleep logs can include such elements as when you went to bed and when you woke up, how many waking periods you had, the quality of dreams ranked from 1 (poor) to 5 (very good), and the quality of sleep ranked from 1 (poor) to 5 (very good). Other elements that may be tracked include naps, time you ate dinner, exercise, and frequency and times of taking sleep medication, drinking alcohol, and smoking.

Example: Identify, over several days, the times to bed and arising, waking periods, dream quality (1–5), and sleep quality (1–5).

EXAMPLE SLEEP LOG

Day	Time to Bed	Time Arising	Nap?	Waking Period(s)	Dream Quality (1–5)	Sleep Quality (1–5)
1	11:00 PM	4:00 AM	Y	12:30–12:35 AM	2	2 (nightmare)
2	10:00 PM	5:00 AM	N	12:30–12:45 AM	3 (practiced image rehearsal therapy)	4
3	10:00 PM	5:00 AM	N	12:30–12:35 AM	4	4
4	10:00 PM	5:30 AM	N	None	4	5

Fig. 3–7. Sleep log example

Identify causes of sleep problems

Weight gained per calorie increases when sleep is disrupted and the natural circadian rhythm is in disarray. The circadian rhythm is the cycle of activity based on a 24-hour period and is influenced by regular variations of night and day. It is this biological clock of sleeping and waking that allows you, for example, to wake around the same time every day even without an alarm clock. But when this rhythm is disrupted, and is made even worse by stress, the overall effect tends to decrease one's metabolism and increase the desire for high caloric food.[66]

We all have beliefs about what it means to have good sleep. For many of us, the ideal night's sleep might be eight dream-filled hours of uninterrupted slumber. Some people, however, suffer from an inability to achieve either the quality or quantity of sleep that they desire. There are both physical and psychological reasons for poor sleep. Certainly, physical pain can disrupt sleep, as can worrying about past or upcoming events. Nightmares or bad dreams can also disrupt sleep.

While sleep-related problems can be associated with work and lifestyle, it is also important to recognize that some sleep problems may be the result of certain medical, neurological, or psychiatric disorders. Sleep-disordered breathing (SDB) and especially sleep apnea, for example, can have an effect on mood and anxiety and can present as attention deficit disorder or even not being able to stay awake in nonstimulating situations. Some of the symptoms of SDB can be loud snoring with frequent awakenings, waking up gasping, morning headache, frequent urination during sleep periods, and dry mouth in the morning.[67,68] Certainly, in this case, we need to reach out to our medical provider.

Aside from changing your thinking about what constitutes sleep, consider the following behaviors or habits you can develop before going to bed.[69,70] Remember to allow yourself approximately two weeks in order to establish a new behavior.

- As adults, remember your bed is for two activities: sleep and sex. Do not read, watch TV, or do anything else in bed.

- Avoid caffeine, cigarettes, and alcohol. The reason for avoiding caffeine and smoking is obvious, but many people think that having a few drinks before bed helps them get to sleep. Studies show that alcohol actually does not help us sleep.[71,72] Being passed out is not the same as being asleep because the deep beneficial levels of sleep do not occur.

- Approximately 20 to 60 minutes before bed, make a purposeful effort to slow down. Do not watch anything on TV that will agitate you. Watching the 10 o'clock news and then trying to go to sleep has never worked well for me; how about you? Do not talk with anyone on the phone where an upset might occur. Do not study for a test right up until bedtime. Spend time listening to soothing music and practice one of your relaxation skills.

- If you are not asleep within 15 to 20 minutes, get out of bed and go watch a boring TV show, read a boring book, play solitaire, or consider some nonstressful activity until you become sleepy. When you are sleepy, return to bed. Repeat the process if needed.

- Sleep in a room that is cool and dark.

- After you have established a baseline and a good sleep pattern using the sleep log, avoid looking at your clock when you wake up in the night.

- Practice positive imagery. The classic lemon exercise demonstrates the effectiveness of this technique. Allow yourself to imagine that you are holding a lemon in your hands. Imagine that you are rubbing the lemon with your thumbs. Feel the texture of the surface of the lemon and notice the crevices and lumps on the skin. Begin to press a little harder on the skin, so that you smell the scent of lemon oil. Continue to rub the lemon with your thumbs and sense the texture and smell of the lemon. Using your thumbs, tear into the lemon. Feel the juice from the lemon as it runs into your hands, and down your wrists and your forearms. The smell and tang of lemon becomes so much more intense. Now, take a bite out of one of the pieces of the lemon. Are you salivating (even though the lemon is imaginary)? Practicing positive imagery and using one of the relaxations skills is a positive sleep hygiene habit.

- Practice gratitude. As you prepare for sleep, rather than just reviewing your day through the lens of what you should have done or what you didn't complete, take time to consider your successes throughout the day, no matter how small. Also, contemplate five things that you are grateful for. Which lens will help you fall asleep?

- When possible, get up at the same time every day.

- Avoid naps, especially in the late afternoon, and limit them to 45 minutes maximum.

- Make your bed each morning. This simple activity will reward you immediately by seeing order, at bedtime by having a neat bed and experiencing a sense of order, and finally, even if the rest of the day goes completely south, your day will not be a total bust because at least you made your bed.

Nightmares

I have had dreams and I have had nightmares,
but I conquered my nightmares because of my dreams.

— Jonas Salk

Research shows that approximately 5% of the population will suffer from nightmares at any given time, but the rates are 50 to 88% higher for trauma survivors.[73,74] Nightmares can be a persistent problem for trauma survivors. First responders or emergency service workers exposed to trauma, or to secondary exposure through trauma victims, can also be affected and react in a manner that is reflective of a trauma victim. This reaction can range from the extreme, in the form of PTSD, to something less symptomatic whereby work seems to take over life in a manner similar to the concept of burnout. In these situations nightmares can and often do become more frequent. These nightmares can be disturbing and can initiate harmful sleep habits, such as using excessive amounts of alcohol and pharmaceuticals in an attempt to anesthetize oneself. Nightmares are not unique to just those who work with trauma, but can significantly impact college students as well.

If the last thought you have before finally going to sleep is "I sure hope I don't have that nightmare," what are the probabilities that you will have that nightmare?

A concrete example of this is as follows: Take a moment to think about anything you want to, whether positive or negative. It doesn't really matter. Just allow any thoughts that you have come to your mind. Any thought at all, but *do not* think about your left hand. *Do not* think about your left hand! You are free to have any thoughts you want, as long as you *do not* think about your left hand! Most of us will struggle to think of anything else, but the reality is most of us end up focused on our left hand.

For example, trauma survivors may avoid going to bed for fear of having nightmares about their trauma. Unfortunately, by avoiding sleep we can increase the likelihood of having those very nightmares. While the actual traumatic event is horrifying, it is important to realize that any subsequent nightmares can be thought of as a series of images. These terrifying images may be still pictures or perhaps something like a movie, but the good news is we can learn to control the images.

Case study: An ER nurse has a persistent nightmare about traumatic injuries from a multiple car accident. The nurse would replay this scene over and over. There would be other days when the nurse would actively block out any thoughts of that call, hoping to avoid remembering the horror of that moment. The nurse would use drugs and alcohol to self-anesthetize after nights of not sleeping for fear of the nightmare returning. Then the nurse learned of the ability to change the nightmare into a dream through a process called image rehearsal training (IRT). As a group discussion and to familiarize ourselves with the sleep log worksheet, how might we develop the nurse's baseline measures (fig. 3–8)?

Identify, over several days, the times to bed and arising, waking periods, dream quality (1–5), and sleep quality (1–5).

ER NURSE'S SLEEP LOG

Day	Time to Bed	Time Arising	Nap?	Waking Period(s)	Dream Quality (1–5)	Sleep Quality (1–5)
1	11:00 PM	4:00 AM	Y	12:30–12:35 AM	2	2 (nightmare)
2	10:00 PM	5:00 AM	N	12:30–12:45 AM	3	4
3	10:00 PM	5:00 AM	N	12:30–12:35 AM	4	4
4	10:00 PM	5:30 AM	N	None	4	5

Fig. 3–8. ER nurse's sleep log

Image rehearsal training is a process of redirecting a bad dream sequence into something more controlled and pleasant:

- Increase your ability to use pleasant images. When we have been traumatized we tend to get really good at visualizing bad things. So, before continuing the exercise, consider spending some time just imagining pleasant things. These can be colors, places, people, or events. Practice this skill several times a day. If you see something pleasurable, stop for a moment and get a picture of that in your mind. Or, you may want to sit quietly for a few minutes and close your eyes and practice getting pleasurable images in your mind, using your senses to fully explore these images or thoughts.

- Choose one bad dream of lower intensity. Write one short paragraph about the scene in first-person, present tense. There is no need to go into extensive detail.

- Change the dream in any way you wish. It is important that some element of the original dream remains intact so that your brain can make the connection with the new change. Write about the changed dream to include information about colors, smells, noises, and anything you can incorporate to increase the vividness of the imagery. You are basically scripting a new movie.

- Finally, form an image of the new dream. Practice by focusing on the new image every day. Along with your sleep habits, log your practice and the effect of the imaging on the nightmare.

Special note: If problems persist you may want to see a psychologist for more in-depth training. Other resources include www.nightmaretreatment.com and www.sleepdynamictherapy.com.

What is the basis for using this technique of imaging? Figure 3–9 illustrates we have what can be referred to as a human imagery system.[75,76]

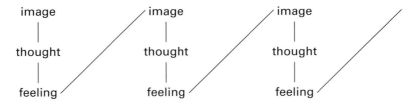

Fig. 3–9. Flow of image, thought, and feeling

Thus, before we have the offensive thought or experience the feeling, we work to interrupt the cycle by implanting a desirable picture or image in our mind.

Reflect: Do you have a recurring nightmare? Practice every day with your newly developed image. Along with your sleep habits, log your practice and the effects from the imaging (fig. 3–10).

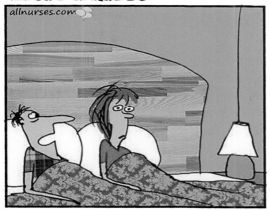

About a Nurse

allnurses.com

"You were nursing in your sleep again. You checked my vitals, gave me an imaginary shot, then mumbled something about doing paperwork."

Fig. 3–10. Dreams can affect our health. (Courtesy allnurses.com.)

INTERNALIZE SLEEP

Sleep is the best meditation.

— Dalai Lama

Think of a time in your life where you were able to get good, quality sleep—not necessarily quantity of sleep, but restful, re-energizing sleep. What were the things you were doing an hour before you went to bed? What things were you thinking about as you got ready for, and as you got into bed? Was the bed made? Was the room cool and completely dark? What do you recall feeling like when you woke up? Write these memories down, as they will help you recall them later and give you clues on how to improve your sleep now.

_____

_____

_____

_____

EXTERNALIZE SLEEP

Insomnia is a gross feeder. It will nourish itself on any kind of thinking, including thinking about not thinking.

— Clifton Fadiman

A number of processes have been examined above to address sleep and sleep-related problems. Given these tools, examine the following case study.

Case study: Unfortunately, severe weather and a tornado had caused damage and injury to your community last year. Several days ago, a series of severe storms again spawned a tornado. Fortunately, the tornado did not cause any damage and passed far from your community. The weather at this time is quite nice and there are no threats of storms. You come across a friend sitting on the curb, under a tree. You stop to ask if the friend is okay. The friend says all is fine but has had trouble sleeping the last few nights since the storms passed through. The friend mentions recurring nightmares about a tornado and asks how you have been sleeping since the storms. The friend mentions a desire to get a good night's sleep. How would you react to this situation and what intervention would you suggest?

_____

_____

_____

_____

PRACTICING SLEEP

Think about how you can best incorporate the concept of sleep into your life today. Specifically, consider a sleep plan to improve your quality of sleep. You may need to pick one or two suggestions to start with. Some recommendations will have an immediate impact and I would urge you try those first. For example, follow the suggestions of turning off your TV 30 minutes before bedtime, practicing a relaxation skill, and avoiding caffeine in the evening.

What recommendations are you going to employ for the next several weeks? Why?

_____

_____

_____

_____

COMMUNITY SLEEP

We've reviewed the downside of poor sleep habits, which can also have a profoundly negative impact on you and your community. I am reminded of a training session with first responders and their families who talked at length of the problems associated poor sleep on their family life. A spouse coming home from a long shift, with little to no sleep, is not a welcome sight to a family. And, if the family has demands for the person coming home, the family is likewise not a welcome sight. Through these exercises the first responders and their families were able to explore the skills and come up with creative solutions to avoid a grizzly bear coming through the door (fig. 3–11). How can you and your support system implement healthy sleep hygiene?

_____

_____

_____

_____

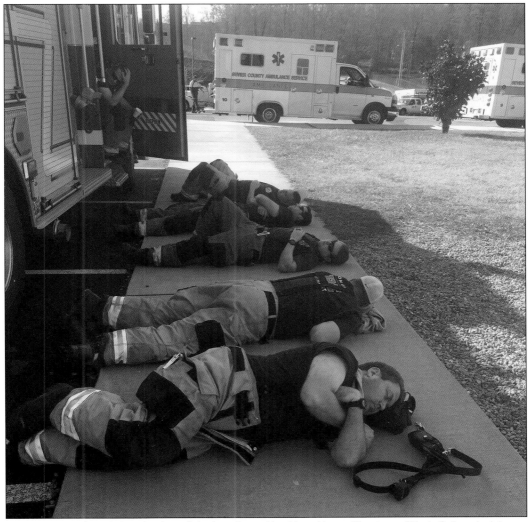

Fig. 3–11. Lack of good sleep has been linked to a host of health problems. (Courtesy of Kevin Colbaugh, Johnson City, TN Fire Department.)

Sleep is the golden chain that ties health and our bodies together.

—Thomas Dekker

REMEMBERING SLEEP

Over the years of teaching this curriculum to veterans, first responders, medical caregivers, and students, the most memorable take away from this skill is (yes you guessed it): "Your bed is for two things and two things only: sleep and sex."

NOTES

1   Jacobson, Edmund. *Progressive Relaxation: A Physiological and Clinical Investigation of Muscular States and their Significance in Psychology and Medical Practice.* Chicago: University of Chicago Press, 1938.

2   Field, Tiffany. "Progressive muscle relaxation." In *Complementary and Alternative Therapies Research.* Washington, DC: American Psychological Association, 2009.

3   Leitch, Laurie and Loree Sutton. *Social Resilience Model (SRM) Level 1 Training.* Brooklyn, NY: Threshold GlobalWorks, 2013, 2-83.

4   Brantley, Jeffrey. "Mindfulness-based stress reduction." In Orsillo, Susan M. and Lizabeth Roemer. *Acceptance- and Mindfulness-based Approaches to Anxiety: Conceptualization and Treatment.* New York: Springer, 2005, 131-145.

5   Kabat-Zinn, Jon. *Mindfulness for Beginners: Reclaiming the Present Moment—and Your Life.* Boulder, CO: Sounds True, Inc., 2012.

6   Shapiro, Shauna L., Kirk Warren Brown, and Gina M. Biegel. "Teaching self-care to caregivers: Effects of mindfulness-based stress reduction on the mental health of therapists in training." *Training and Education in Professional Psychology* 1, no. 2 (2007): 105.

7   Sapolsky, Robert M. *Why Zebras Don't Get Ulcers: The Acclaimed Guide to Stress, Stress-related Diseases, and Coping.* New York: Henry Holt and Co., 2004.

8   Lupien, Sonia J., Bruce S. McEwen, Megan R. Gunnar, and Christine Heim. "Effects of stress throughout the lifespan on the brain, behaviour and cognition." *Nature Reviews Neuroscience* 10, no. 6 (2009): 434-445.

9   Lovallo, William R. *Stress and Health: Biological and Psychological Interactions.* Thousand Oaks, CA: Sage Publications, 2015.

10 Boscarino, Joseph A. "Posttraumatic stress disorder and physical illness: Results from clinical and epidemiologic studies." *Annals of the New York Academy of Sciences* 1032, no. 1 (2004): 141-153.

11 Pacella, Maria L., Bryce Hruska, and Douglas L. Delahanty. "The physical health consequences of PTSD and PTSD symptoms: A meta-analytic review." *Journal of Anxiety Disorders* 27, no. 1 (2013): 33-46.

12 Schnurr, Paula P. and Bonnie L. Green, eds. *Trauma and Health: Physical Health Consequences of Exposure to Extreme Stress.* Washington, DC: American Psychological Association, 2004.

13 Cohen, Sheldon. "Social relationships and health." *American Psychologist* 59, no. 8 (2004): 676-684.

14 American Psychological Association. "Stress in America: Paying with Our Health, 2015." https://www.apa.org/news/press/releases/stress/2014/stress-report.pdf.

15 Wharton University of Pennsylvania. "Reluctant vacationers: Why Americans work more, relax less, than Europeans." http://knowledge.wharton.upenn.edu/article/reluctant-vacationers-why-americans-work-more-relax-less-than-europeans/.

16 Centers for Disease Control and Prevention (CDC). "Perceived insufficient rest or sleep among adults—United States, 2008." *MMWR Morbidity and Mortality Weekly Report* 58, no. 42 (2009): 1175.

17 Gunderson, Johathan, Mike Grill, Phillip Callahan, and Michael Marks. "An evidence-based program for improving and sustaining first responder behavioral health." *Journal of Emergency Medical Services* (2014): 57-61.

18 Institute of Medicine. *Sleep Disorders and Sleep Deprivation: An Unmet Public Health Problem.* Washington, DC: The National Academies Press, 2006.

19 Wu, Joseph C., Monte Buchsbaum, and William E. Bunney. "Clinical neurochemical implications of sleep deprivation's effects on the anterior cingulate of depressed responders." *Neuropsychopharmacology* 25, suppl. 5 (2001): S74-S78.

20 Greer, Stephanie M., Andrea N. Goldstein, and Matthew P. Walker. "The impact of sleep deprivation on food desire in the human brain." *Nature Communications* 4 (2013) 2259.

21 Wolf, Lisa A., Cydne Perhats, Altair Delao, and Zoran Martinovich. "The effect of reported sleep, perceived fatigue, and sleepiness on cognitive performance in a sample of emergency nurses." *Journal of Nursing Administration* 47, no. 1 (2017): 41-49.

22 Thomas, Cynthia M., Constance E. McIntosh, Ruth Ann Lamar, and Roberta L. Allen. "Sleep deprivation in nursing students: The negative impact for quality and safety." *Journal of Nursing Education and Practice* 7, no. 5 (2017): 87.

23 Carter, Briana, Joanne Chopak-Foss, and Fadzai B. Punungwe. "An analysis of the sleep quality of undergraduate students." *College Student Journal* 50, no. 3 (2016): 315-322.

24 Walker, Anthony, Andrew McKune, Sally Ferguson, David B. Pyne, and Ben Rattray. "Chronic occupational exposures can influence the rate of PTSD and depressive disorders in first responders and military personnel." *Extreme Physiology & Medicine* 5, no. 1 (2016): 8.

25   Pelletier, Cori L. "The effect of music on decreasing arousal due to stress: A meta-analysis." *Journal of Music Therapy* 41, no. 3 (2004): 192-214.

26   Cooper, John O., Timothy E. Heron, and William L. Heward. *Applied Behavior Analysis*. Upper Saddle River, NJ: Pearson, 2007, 37-46.

27   Lambert, Michael J. *Bergin and Garfield's Handbook of Psychotherapy and Behavior Change*. Hoboken, NJ: John Wiley & Sons, 2013.

28   Sullivan, Alycia N. and Margie E. Lachman. "Behavior change with fitness technology in sedentary adults: A review of the evidence for increasing physical activity." *Frontiers in Public Health* 4, no. 289 (2017): 1.

29   Cahalin, Lawrence P., Malinda Braga, Yoshimi Matsuo, and Edgar D. Hernandez. "Efficacy of diaphragmatic breathing in persons with chronic obstructive pulmonary disease: A review of the literature." *Journal of Cardiopulmonary Rehabilitation and Prevention* 22, no. 1 (2002): 7-21.

30   Martarelli, Daniele, Mario Cocchioni, Stefania Scuri, and Pierluigi Pompei. "Diaphragmatic breathing reduces exercise-induced oxidative stress." *Evidence-Based Complementary and Alternative Medicine* (2011): 932430.

31   Upadhyay, Dhungel, K., V. Malhotra, D. Sarkar, and R. Prajapati. "Effect of alternate nostril breathing exercise on cardiorespiratory functions." *Nepal Medical College Journal* 10, no. 1 (2008): 25-27.

32   Bernstein, Douglas A., Thomas D. Borkovec, and Holly Hazlett-Stevens. *New Directions in Progressive Relaxation Training: A Guidebook for Helping Professionals*. Westport, CT: Praeger Press, 2000, 5-24.

33   Davis, Martha, Elizabeth Robbins Eshelman, and Matthew McKay. *The Relaxation and Stress Reduction Workbook*. Oakland CA: Harbinger Publications, 2008, 41-46.

34   Coffey, Scott F., Julie A. Schumacher, Marcella L. Brimo, and Kathleen T. Brady. "Exposure therapy for substance abusers with PTSD: Translating research to practice." *Behavior Modification* 29, no. 1 (2005): 10-38.

35   Kabat-Zinn, Jon. *Wherever You Go, There You Are: Mindfulness Meditation in Everyday Life*. New York: Hyperion, 1994, 3-8.

36   Kabat-Zinn, Jon. *Coming to Our Senses: Healing Ourselves and the World Through Mindfulness*. New York: Hyperion, 2005, 19-114.

37   Stahl, Bob and Elisha Goldstein. *A Mindfulness-based Stress Reduction Workbook*. Oakland, CA: New Harbinger, 2010, 191-198.

38   Siegel, Daniel J. *The Mindful Brain: Reflection and Attunement in the Cultivation of Well-Being*. New York: W.W. Norton, 2007, 3-30.

39   Grossman, Paul, Ludger Niemann, Stefan Schmidt, and Harald Walach. "Mindfulness-based stress reduction and health benefits: A meta-analysis." *Journal of Psychosomatic Research* 57, no. 1 (2004): 35-43.

40   Carmody, James, George Reed, Jean Kristeller, and Phillip Merriam. "Mindfulness, spirituality, and health-related symptoms." *Journal of Psychosomatic Research* 64, no. 4 (2008): 393-403.

41   Halford, Scott G. *Activate Your Brain: How Understanding Your Brain Can Improve Your Work—and Your Life*. Austin, TX: Greenleaf Book Group Press, 2015.

42   Hölzel, Britta K., James Carmody, Mark Vangel, Christina Congleton, Sita M. Yerramsetti, Tim Gard, and Sara W. Lazar. "Mindfulness practice leads to increases in regional brain gray matter density." *Psychiatry Research: Neuroimaging* 191, no. 1 (2011): 36-43.

43   Copeland, Mary Ellen. "Wellness recovery action plan: A system for monitoring, reducing and eliminating uncomfortable or dangerous physical symptoms and emotional feelings." *Occupational Therapy in Mental Health* 17, no. 3-4 (2002): 127-150.

44   Lingner, H., B. Burger, P. Kardos, C. P. Criée, H. Worth, and E. Hummers-Pradier. "What patients really think about asthma guidelines: Barriers to guideline implementation from the patients' perspective." *BMC Pulmonary Medicine* 17, no. 1 (2017): 13.

45   Holloway, Elizabeth A. and Robert J. West. "Integrated breathing and relaxation training (the Papworth method) for adults with asthma in primary care: A randomised controlled trial." *Thorax* 62, no. 12 (2007): 1039-1042.

46   Alexander, A. Barney, Gerd J. A. Cropp, and Hyman Chai. "Effects of relaxation training on pulmonary mechanics in children with asthma." *Journal of Applied Behavior Analysis* 12, no. 1 (1979): 27-35.

47   Schutz, Paul A. and Heather A. Davis. "Emotions and self-regulation during test taking." *Educational Psychologist* 35, no. 4 (2000): 243-256.

48   Davis, Heather A., Christine DiStefano, and Paul A. Schutz. "Identifying patterns of appraising tests in first-year college students: Implications for anxiety and emotion regulation during test taking." *Journal of Educational Psychology* 100, no. 4 (2008): 942-960.

49   Elliot, Diane L. and Kerry S. Kuehl. *Effects of Sleep Deprivation on Fire Fighters and EMS Responders: Final Report, June 2007*. Fairfax, VA: International Association of Fire Chiefs (IAFC) and the United States Fire Administration (USFA), 2007. https://www.iafc.org/docs/default-source/uploaded-documents/progssleep-sleepdeprivationreport.pdf.

50   Ferrie, Jane E. Martin J. Shipley, Francesco P. Cappuccio, Erc Brunner, Michelle A. Miller, Meena Kumari, and Michael G. Marmot. "A prospective study of change in sleep duration: Associations with mortality in the Whitehall II cohort." *Sleep* 30, no. 12 (2007): 1659-1666.

51   Curcio, Giuseppe, Michele Ferrara, and Luigi De Gennaro. "Sleep loss, learning capacity and academic performance." *Sleep Medicine Review* 10 no. 5 (2006): 323-337.

52   Medeiros, Ana L. D., Denise B. F. Mendes, Patricia F. Lima, and John F. Araujo. "The relationships between sleep-wake cycle and academic performance in medical students." *Biological Rhythm Research* 32, no. 2 (2001): 263-270.

53   Spiegel, Karine, Rachel Leproult, and Eve Van Cauter. "Impact of sleep debt on metabolic and endocrine function." *The Lancet* 354, no. 9188 (1999): 1435-1439.

54   Harrison, Yvonne and James A. Horne. "The impact of sleep deprivation on decision making: A review." *Journal of Experimental Psychology: Applied* 6, no. 3 (2000): 236-239.

55   Gaultney, Jane F. "The prevalence of sleep disorders in college students: Impact on academic performance." *Journal of American College Health* 59, no. 2 (2010): 91-97.

56   Elliot, Diane L. and Kerry S. Kuehl. *Effects of Sleep Deprivation on Fire Fighters and EMS Responders: Final Report, June 2007*. Fairfax, VA: International Association of Fire Chiefs (IAFC) and the United States Fire Administration (USFA), 2007. https://www.iafc.org/docs/default-source/uploaded-documents/progssleep-sleepdeprivationreport.pdf.

57   Ibid.

58   Curcio, Giuseppe, Michele Ferrara, and Luigi De Gennaro. "Sleep loss, learning capacity and academic performance." *Sleep Medicine Review* 10 no. 5 (2006): 323-337.

59   Medeiros, Ana L. D., Denise B. F. Mendes, Patricia F. Lima, and John F. Araujo. "The relationships between sleep-wake cycle and academic performance in medical students." *Biological Rhythm Research* 32, no. 2 (2001): 263-270.

60   Buboltz Jr., Walter, Steve M. Jenkins, Barlow Soper, Kevin Woller, Patrick Johnson, and Theresa Faes. "Sleep habits and patterns of college students: An expanded study." *Journal of College Counseling* 12, no. 2 (2009): 113-124.

61   Thacher, Pamela V. "University students and 'the all nighter': Correlates and patterns of students' engagement in a single night of total sleep deprivation." *Behavioral Sleep Medicine* 6, no. 1 (2008): 16-31.

62   Gresham, Samuel C., Wilse B. Webb, and Robert L. Williams. "Alcohol and caffeine: Effect on inferred visual dreaming." *Science* 140, no. 3572 (1963): 1226-1227.

63   Yules, Richard B., Marc E. Lippman, and Daniel X. Freedman. "Alcohol administration prior to sleep: The effect on EEG sleep stage." *Archives of General Psychiatry* 16, no. 1 (1967): 94-97.

64   Peeke, Shirley C., Enoch Callaway, Reese T. Jones, George C. Stone, and Joseph Doyle. "Combined effects of alcohol and sleep deprivation in normal young adults." *Psychopharmacology* 67 no. 3 (1980): 279-287.

65   Drew, Liam. "What is the point of sleep?" *New Scientist* 217, no. 2902 (2013): 38-39.

66   Gamble, Jessa. "The sleep squeeze." *New Scientist* 217, no. 2902 (2013): 34-37.

67   Doghramji, Karl. "Clinical features of sleep-disordered breathing." *Psychiatric Times* (Feb 4, 2014). http://www.psychiatrictimes.com/sleep-disorders/clinical-features-sleep-disordered-breathing.

68   Bootzin, Richard R. Diana Epstine, James M. Wood. "Stimulus Control Instructions." In Hauri, Peter J., ed. *Case Studies in Insomnia*. New York: Plenum Medical Book, 1991, 19-28.

69   Edinger, Jack D. and Colleen E. Carney. *Overcoming Insomnia: A Cognitive Behavioral Therapy Approach*. Oxford, NY: Oxford University Press, 2008, 7-10.

70   Perlis, Michael L., Carla Jungquist, Michael T. Smith, Donn Posner. *Cognitive Behavioral Treatment of Insomnia: A Session-by-Session Guide*. New York: Springer, 2005, 12-24.

71   Bonnet, Michale H. and Donna L. Arand. "We are chronically sleep deprived," *Sleep* 18, no. 10 (1995): 908-911.

72   Perlis, Michael L., Carla Jungquist, Michael T. Smith, and Donn Posner. *Cognitive Behavioral Treatment of Insomnia: A Session-by-Session Guide*. New York: Springer, 2005, 12-24.

73   Bixler, Edward, A. Kales, C. R. Soldatos, J. D. Kales, and S. Healey. "Prevalence of sleep disorders in the Los Angeles metropolitan area." *American Journal of Psychiatry* 136, no. 10 (1979): 1257-1262.

74   Krakow, Barry and Antonio Zadra. "Clinical management of chronic nightmares: Imagery rehearsal therapy." *Behavioral Sleep Medicine* 4, no. 1 (2006): 45-70.

75   van Schagen, Annette M., Japp Lancee, Victor I. Spoormaker, and Jan van den Bout. "Long-term treatment effects of imagery rehearsal therapy for nightmares in a population with diverse psychiatric disorders." *International Journal of Dream Research* 9, no. 1 (2016): 67-70.

76   Krakow, Barry. "Nightmare therapy: Emerging concepts from sleep medicine." In Kramer, Milton and Myron Glucksman, eds. *Dream Research: Contributions to Clinical Practice*. New York: Routledge, 2015, 149.

4

PERSPECTIVE

Some people see the glass half full. Others see it half empty.
I see a glass that's twice as big as it needs to be.

— George Carlin

OVERVIEW

Why: One of the more powerful ways to reduce stress is to change the way an event is perceived.

How: Accept the situation that confronts you with a realistic view, without minimizing, exaggerating, or catastrophizing. Recognize, too, that while the present situation may not be changeable, a change of attitude is possible. Following are some steps that can be used to modify your perspective:

- Identify the stressor(s) and the associated worst fear(s).
- Explore what beliefs confine you to those thoughts.
- Consider an alternative, more attractive consequence.
- Identify what you can do to encourage this option.
- Attune your beliefs to conform with your realigned objective.
- Recognize that the stressor or situation may not be changeable, but remember that you are.

Identifying a measure of change between before and after developing the goal and steps to meet the goal provides us a measure of our success. We use the Subjective Units of Distress Scale (SUDS) to help subjectively identify your stress level before, and again after, as somewhere between zero (0) and ten (10), where 0 corresponds to no stress and 10 to the highest level of stress you have ever experienced. The anticipation is that the SUDS level begins to decrease even after developing a goal statement and the steps to attain the goal. If your SUDS level increases, take some time to reassess the goal statement to assure it is attainable. And reassess the steps to assure that they have been adequately defined and there are a sufficient number. After all, you want to be able to check off each step and mark progress toward reaching your goal.

Goal Setting Skill—Perspective

Challenging our old ways of seeing ourselves, others, and the world takes courage. Remember courage is not the absence of stress or fear.

Rate the stress level you perceive

Analog SUDS	Digital SUDS	Emoji SUDS
Actually, I'm not stressed	0	
A little stressed	1–3	
Somewhat stressed	4–6	
Quite a bit stressed	7–8	
It's really bad	9	
Run and hide!!	10	

Think about what's stressing you out. What might help?

Try and identify an objective to help you do that.

Now it's time to figure out how you can get there.

Write out a goal statement about how you might look at your dilemmas differently.

Now, how do you plan to get there, step-by-step?

Now get started! Don't be shy. Go for it!

Have you made any progress?

Rate the stress level you perceive now

Is it lower?

Yes	No
  Congratulations!! You did it!! Now you can do this whenever you need it!	What might have gone wrong? Did you figure out all your steps? Did you actually do them all? Did you earmark enough time to ponder? Were your reflections satisfying? Are you impatient and haven't allowed enough time to see change? Give it another try, from the beginning.

Is SUDS the only option for measuring change? Certainly not! You are encouraged to find the most appropriate measurement for your needs. The only thing that matters is that it can provide meaningful feedback with regard to change, or even transformation, resulting from applying the goal-setting process. Perhaps a scale that measures the likelihood of completing the task might be more useful. That scale might range from 0 to 10, where 0 corresponds to zero chance of completion and 10 is fully sure of completion. If you were using a likelihood-of-completion scale, then you would anticipate an increase in likelihood to complete from premeasure to postmeasure.

WHY PERSPECTIVE?

William James, the 19th century American physician and philosopher considered by many to be the father of American psychology, once said that "the greatest discovery of my generation was that a person could alter their lives by altering their attitude."

It's still true in the 21st century. One of the most powerful ways we can reduce our stress is to change our perspective about the stresses that confront us. This is not say that we have our heads in the clouds or have a "Don't worry! Be happy!" attitude toward everything that happens to us. Or that we are always the stoic "Suck it up, ruck it up, drive on!" type. Sometimes… sometimes life sucks!! And resilient people know that. At the same time, we don't want to exaggerate or catastrophize every stressful situation that confronts us. Doing any of these extremes limits our problem-solving skills, erodes our self-efficacy, and impairs our ability to be resilient.

If we perceive a predicament as a matter of life and death, we will likely act much differently than if we see the context as temporary or unlikely to cause any lasting harm. A way to modify our perception is to modify our pattern of thought or our perspective of the dilemma. In doing so, we alter the way in which we respond to a potentially stressful situation and are therefore able to assess the context more accurately.[1] Perspective helps us to methodically resolve a problematic puzzle and not become part of it. In fact, we can become prisoners of our own thoughts and perspectives.[2,3] To break free of these we must strive to assess the circumstances as objectively as possible, avoiding the traps of self-defeating thought patterns.

> *If you'll recall, at the beginning of this text I pointed out that one of the challenges you will face on this journey to becoming more resilient is to honestly confront your biases, stereotypes, and self-defeating thought patterns. Relax, we all have them.*

While we have been exploring some of the more behavioral and physical skills of resilience,[4] it's now time to look at what goes on between our ears: our cognitions and perceptions. Cognitions are those mental things that either promote our resilience or become obstacles to our growth, our ability to cope, and to help those around us.

One aspect of perspective is emotional intelligence.[5] This is a cognitive skill that will be important as we explore the remainder of the resilience skills. The good news is that it is a skill that can be taught and learned, and is recognized as just as important in success as our IQ.[6] *Emotional intelligence* has many definitions, but is best understood as the ability to identify our own emotions and those of others. It is also the ability to channel those emotions and make them work for us as we attempt to solve problems (fig. 4–1). Emotional intelligence, or EI, is also the ability to manage emotions, both in ourselves and others.[7,8]

How good are you at calming down others or cheering someone up? How comfortable are you allowing someone to grieve? If you are a first responder being called to a multiple car accident, are you able to accurately recognize your emotions or have you learned to numb-out and run through your protocol without any emotion? The latter becomes a foot in the door to developing PTSD. As a student, do you become paralyzed with fear before a test rather than recognizing that your anxiety is a call to action?

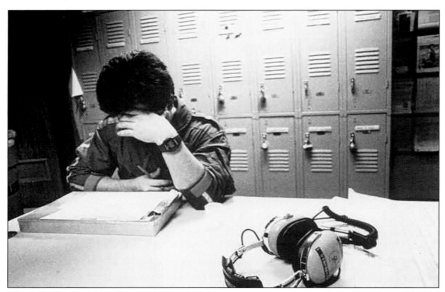

Fig. 4–1. Emotional intelligence is the ability to manage our own emotions. (Courtesy of Mike Grill.)

Perspective can have a profound impact on how we cope with significant events in our lives and their aftermath. Professor Warren Bennis was the youngest infantry commander in the European theater during WWII and earned a Bronze Star and Purple Heart for his bravery. After the war, he returned to college, eventually earning a Ph.D. from MIT. From there he became an international icon in the field of leadership. Professor Bennis espoused the notion of *servant leadership*, where leaders view themselves as being there to assist, support, encourage, and inspire their followers to achieve their common goal.[9,10] Simon Sinek, a popular author and motivational speaker, has a stirring talk about servant leadership entitled *Why Leaders Eat Last*.[11] Bennis, from his own experiences and studying leadership styles, recognized that all leaders must endure a crucible event.[12,13] Crucible events are the experiences that test us and force us to question ourselves and what matters to us. In our leadership class, we ask student veterans to write about a crucible event in their lives and how it has impacted their leadership style. Of course, most will write about some event during their time in war and are often fond of the old refrain, "I wouldn't give a penny to do it again, but I wouldn't take a million dollars for the experience." It is that perspective that allows them to integrate those life-changing events into their lives in a positive way.

A relatively small field of study has emerged called *post-traumatic growth*. Its proponents theorize that we do not need to be victims of the tragedies that befall us, but that we can become survivors and, in fact, grow and become better people because of those events.[14,15] For example, a study found that 61% of the aviators who were shot down, imprisoned, and tortured by the North Vietnamese noted psychological benefits from their ordeals.[16]

To achieve such a psychological feat in our own lives requires us to have a flexible mindset, as compared to a fixed state of mind.[17,18,19] Research has shown that people with flexible attitudes or sets of opinions are better able to cope with stress compared with those who have rigid attitudes.[20,21] Fortunately, we can learn to have a more flexible mind-set, but it requires us to suspend some of our deeply ingrained ways of viewing ourselves, other people, and the world.[22,23]

I ask not for a lighter burden, but for broader shoulders.

— Jewish proverb

THE HOW OF PERSPECTIVE

One of the ways that we can help maximize our resiliency in the face of a stressful situation is to change our perspective about that situation. The process considers the probabilities of the worst case and alternative outcomes.[24,25,26] And, while the stressful situation may be quite dire, we do have the potential to change the way we react to it. Some perceived good can emerge from the struggle. For example, this struggle may yield a change in self-perception, interpersonal relationships, or philosophy of life.[27]

What does perspective mean to you?

_____

_____

_____

_____

Perspective Checklist

Thinking carefully, what do you see as the issue(s) or problem(s) that need to be addressed?

Identify, as best you can, the dilemma:

> What are your fears here?
>
> What is evoking these fears?
>
> How likely do you think the problem(s) will create the feared conclusion(s)?
>
> Do you see this as an adversity?   Why?
>
> Do you see this as an opportunity?   Why?

When you started to review your plans:

> What is your baseline SUDS?
>
> How does this situation fit with what you had thought about before?
>
> Did thinking about this change your SUDS?   Why?

Now, the what, where, and how:

> Think about how you are holding yourself hostage.
>
> What alternative conclusion(s) would you want?
>
> How will you encourage it?
>
> Think about how likely this option might be.
>
> How long will you commit?

After you review the above steps:

> What SUDS level are you enduring now?

Do you think you might use any of our other skills?   Which ones?

Now let's think about whether all this helps:

Will tracking your emerging options generate greater incentive to continue?   Why?

Will tracking your beliefs evolution provide better feedback?   Why?

Did this process make your impression of the event more manageable?   How?

Did this process make your impression of the event more compelling?   How?

Can you think of anything you might change in this skill to make it more personally useful?

How about the future? Do you think you will be able to put your results to the test?

We who lived in concentration camps can remember the men who walked
through the huts comforting others, giving away their last piece of bread.
They may have been few in number, but they offer sufficient
proof that everything can be taken from a man but one thing:
the last of the human freedoms—to choose one's attitude
in any given set of circumstances, to choose one's own way.

—Viktor Frankl

Activity: Following is an example of how to use the worst case and alternative worksheet. Use the case study below and begin to:

- Identify the stressful situation.

- Identify your worst fear or fears.

- Consider how likely it is that these worst fears will come true.

- Identify an alternative scenario or scenarios, potentially more positive, of what is most likely to occur. Even though they may not be able to alter the present situation, the alternative(s) may include consideration about how we as individuals can grow as a consequence.

- Don't ignore the fact that stressful and traumatic events can evoke positive psychological changes.[28]

- Identify any needs you will have to gather together to help make a substitute scenario come true.

- Determine what is the likelihood that this alternative outcome will come true.

I've had many catastrophes in my life, some of which actually happened.

— Mark Twain

Case study: A friend confides in you that his need to work, attend classes, and have a social life is taxing and beginning to wear him down. Wanting to make some advancement at work, he is taking on some work-related studies.

In the midst of all this, your friend is suffering from a recurring stomachache. This has gone on for about three days and was initially attributed to too much fast food. But the condition seems to persist and he is beginning to worry that the stomachache might be something very serious.

As a group discussion and to familiarize ourselves with the perspective worksheet, how might we put this situation into perspective?

Consider using the following checklist as a map or guide for completing this leg of your journey.

Case Study Example Checklist

Thinking carefully, what do you see as the issue(s) and problem(s) that need to be addressed?

Identify, as best you can, the dilemma:

> What are your fears here?
>
> What is evoking these fears?
>
> How likely do you think the problem(s) will create the feared conclusion(s)?
>
> Do you see this as an adversity?   Why?
>
> Do you see this as an opportunity?   Why?

When you start to review your thoughts:

> What is your baseline SUDS level?
>
> How does this situation fit with what you had thought about before?
>
> Did thinking about this change your SUDS level?   Why?

Now, the what, where, and how:

> Think about how you are holding yourself hostage.
>
> What alternative conclusion(s) would you want?
>
> How will you encourage it?
>
> Think about how likely this option might be.
>
> How long will you commit?

After you review these steps:

> What is your resulting SUDS?
>
> Do you think you might use any of our other skills?   Which ones?

Now let's think about whether all this helps:

> Did this process make your impression of the event more manageable?   How?
>
> Did this process make your impression of the event more compelling?   How?

Can you think of anything you might change in this skill to make it more personally useful?

How about the future? Do you think you will be able to put your results to the test?

Our problems are just solutions looking for a home.

— Neil Atkinson

If writing this as narrative, in a story format, the worksheet above can serve as a guide or an example of how this might be done. Remember that writing can be a powerful tool in clarifying, recalling, and integrating the skill into your life.

_____

_____

_____

_____

In the book of life, the answers aren't in the back.

— Charlie Brown

HUMOR

To succeed in life, you need three things:
a wishbone, a backbone, and a funny bone.

— Reba McEntire

Why humor: Humor and the ability to laugh have a number of protective and healing qualities against the effects of stress. Just don't forget that there is often a very distinct flavor of humor associated with our various professions. If an outsider to our profession were to examine the humor that emerges, this outsider might consider it extreme or even off-color.

To be honest, there is humor that I use in the first responder, emergency medical, and veteran communities that I have learned, painfully, to not use in the civilian world. Yet, this humor (properly applied, of course) makes those of us who share these situations laugh and helps to relieve our tension.

Laughter can improve the immune system.[29,30,31] It can relax the entire body.[32] Laughter can protect the heart[33] (fig. 4–2). Finally, humor and laughter release endorphins, which improve our mood and act as natural painkillers.[34,35]

So, please continue to laugh; just make sure you know who your audience is.

Warning: Humor may be hazardous to your illness.

—Ellie Katz

How humor: How important is humor to you in coping with the stresses in life and work? Are you able to laugh at yourself?

Here is a simple exercise to help you understand how humor can be of help to you in your work life. Pick a period of time, perhaps a work shift, and monitor how often you laugh. At the beginning and at the end of the shift, monitor your mood using a SUDS scale. What do the results suggest? Describe how humor helps you cope with the stress of your job.

Humor is the great thing, the saving thing. The minute it crops up, all our
irritations and resentments slip away, and a sunny spirit takes their place.

— Mark Twain

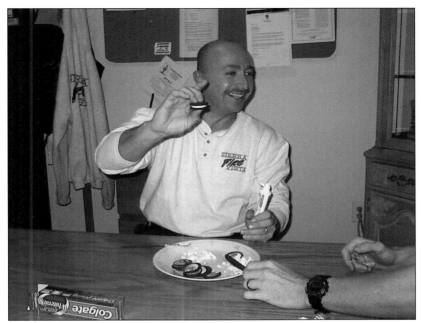

Fig. 4–2. Laughter can improve your immune system. (Courtesy of Mike Grill.)

INTERNALIZING PERSPECTIVE

Perspective helps us to methodically resolve problematic situations. We do this not by becoming part of it, but by mindfully focusing on the present moment and minimizing extraneous, possibly erroneous, thinking. This mindful focus provides us with a means of self-regulation.[36] Having a perspective on a situation can increase our emotional intelligence. As this will increase the likelihood that we can cope with the current stressor, we have a better potential to come up with far more creative solutions to whatever problems we are grappling with.[37,38,39] Many of us have learned, through painful experience, that when we are in the middle of a stressful event we often think that the situation is the worst thing that has ever happened to us.

How: Examining how to put things in perspective can permit more insight into the idea of adjusting and growing beyond the current situation. Again, as with all of our skills, recall, in as much detail as possible, a past personal experience where you used perspective to address a stressful dilemma. The intent is to reflect upon a past experience in sufficient detail to complete all, or as many of the entries, as possible.

I certainly recall how my coronary artery bypass surgery changed my perspective! I was then able to use my crucible events to improve the quality of my life, physically and mentally. In my years of doing trauma therapy, it is when veterans or first responders are able to see an event from a different point of view (perspective) that healing begins. The events do not change, but we do—by looking at ourselves, other people, and the world through a different lens (fig. 4–3). I have friends and colleagues who have taken the horrific events that they have confronted and used them to become some of the best trauma therapists and peer support team members you can find.

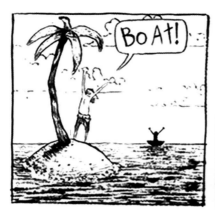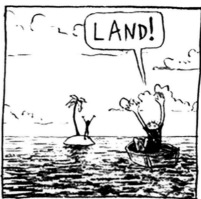

Perspective...

Fig. 4–3. What is your perspective?

Reflect: Use think-aloud pair problem solving (TAPPS) to assist you, as needed, in the following exercise. Recall, in as much detail as possible, a past personal experience where you used perspective to address a stressful situation and complete the entries in the following worksheet.

Checklist for Internalizing Perspective

Thinking carefully, what did you see as the issue(s) and problem(s) that needed to be addressed?

Identify, as best you can, the dilemma:

What were your fears?

What was evoking those fears?

How likely did you think they would create the feared conclusion(s)?

Did you see this as an adversity?   Why?

Did you see this as an opportunity?   Why?

When you start to review your thoughts:

What was your baseline SUDS?

How did this situation fit with what you had thought about before?

Did thinking about this change your SUDS?   Why?

Now, the what, where, and how:

Think about how you were holding yourself hostage.

What alternative conclusion(s) did you want?

How did you encourage it?

Think about how likely this option seemed.

How long did you commit?

After you reviewed these steps, what is your resulting SUDS:

Do you think you might have used any of our other skills?   Which ones?

Now let's think about whether all this helped:

Did this process make your impression of the event more manageable?   How?

Did this process make your impression of the event more compelling?   How?

Can you think of anything you might change in this skill to make it more personally useful?

How about the future? Do you think you will be able to put your results to the test?

Reflect: Recognizing that you have used perspective in the past, do you feel more in control and empowered to address a stressful event?

_____

_____

_____

_____

EXTERNALIZE: APPLY PERSPECTIVE AS A GROUP

To change our perspective about a situation is to consider the probabilities of the worst-case and alternative outcomes. Perspective allows us to grow as a result of an ordeal by using adaptive skills, behaviors, and attitudes developed in response to those circumstances. It reminds us that even trauma survivors are not powerless victims. Given these tools, let's examine the following case study. The intent is to apply the skill to someone other than yourself.

Case study: A fire has devastated several structures, including your neighbor's house. Miraculously, no one was physically injured. Your neighbor, with her two children, is standing in front of the rubble bemoaning the loss of the house. The homeowner looks to you for support. How would you react to this situation and what intervention would you provide?

Reflect: Using TAPPS, develop a possible intervention to the case study in collaborative groups.

Checklist for Externalizing Perspective

Thinking carefully, what do you see as the issue(s) and problem(s) that need to be addressed?

Identify, as best you can, the dilemma:

What are her fears here?

What is evoking these fears?

How likely do you think these problem(s) will create the feared conclusion(s)?

Does she see this as an adversity?   Why?

Does she see this as an opportunity?   Why?

When you start to review your thoughts:

What is her baseline SUDS?

How does this situation fit with what you had thought about before?

Did considering this change her SUDS?   Why?

Now, her what, where, and how:

Think about how she might be holding herself hostage.

What alternative conclusion(s) would you want for her?

How will you encourage it?

Help her think about how likely this option might be.

How long will she commit?

After you reviewed these steps with her, what is her resulting SUDS?

Do you think you might suggest she use any of our other skills?   Which ones?

Now let's think about whether all this helps:

Did this process make her impression of the event more manageable?   How?

Did this process make her impression of the event more compelling?   How?

Can you think of anything you might change in this skill to make it more personally useful?

How about the future? Do you think you will be able to put your results to future tests?

PRACTICE PERSPECTIVE

Think of a situation that you are struggling with in your life right now. How could you best incorporate the concept of perspective into your lifestyle? Specifically, develop a perspective worksheet for a current issue you are facing.

Checklist for Practicing Perspective

Thinking carefully, what do you see as the issue(s) and problem(s) that needed to be addressed?

Identify, as best you can, the dilemma:

What are your fears?

What is evoking those fears?

How likely do you think these will create the feared conclusion(s)?

Do you see this as an adversity?   Why?

Do you see this as an opportunity?   Why?

When you start to review your thoughts:

What is your baseline SUDS?

How did this situation fit with what you had thought about before?

Did thinking about this change your SUDS?   Why?

Now, the what, where, and how:

Think about how you are holding yourself hostage.

What alternative conclusion(s) do you want?

How will you encourage it?

Think about how likely this option seems.

How long will you commit?

After you reviewed these steps, what is your resulting SUDS:

Do you think you might use any of our other skills?   Which ones?

Now let's think about whether all this helped:

Did this process make your impression of the event more manageable?   How?

Did this process make your impression of the event more compelling?   How?

Can you think of anything you might change in this skill to make it more personally useful?

How about the future? Do you think you will be able to put your results to the test?

As before, if writing this as narrative, in a story format, the above guide can be used as an example of how this might be organized.

_____

_____

_____

_____

Reflect: After applying and practicing perspective views, did using the worksheet permit you to develop a more realistic approach to dealing with stressful incidents?

_____

_____

_____

_____

If the only tool you have is a hammer, you tend to see every problem as a nail.

— Abraham Maslow

APPLY PERSPECTIVE TO YOUR COMMUNITY

It is not enough for us to apply the skills just to ourselves. These skills will undoubtedly help us and our communities as we define them. To offer them to our community is to be a mentor to those around us.[40,41]

Consider the following discussion points:

- Define the community where you are intending to apply the skill.

- Why is this skill appropriate for the particular community?

- How would the skill be administered?

- What techniques might you use to introduce the concept of perspective views? What would be your specific expectation of the outcome?

Reflect: How important is it to your community to be able to use perspective views?

> *I am reminded of a training event we did outside Durango, Colorado. As we were taking a break, an elderly gentleman came in and asked if this was the historical society meeting. I explained no, but offered to walk him down to the room where that meeting was being held. As we walked down the hall, I noticed that his ball cap had the Upper Pine River Fire District logo and "CHAPLAIN" across the front. When I inquired, he informed me that he had fought fires in the district for more than 40 years, but that he couldn't fight fires anymore. Then he gently grabbed my arm and with a smile and a twinkle in his eye, he said, "but I can still pray for rain."*
>
> *Now that's perspective!*

If peace comes from seeing the whole,
then misery stems from a loss of perspective.

— Mark Nepo

REMEMBERING PERSPECTIVE

Take the opportunity now to reflect on the skill and associate some key words or phrases that help to succinctly define the skill using your own words. When you have completed this process, compare these key words and phrases with the person or persons with whom you are working. Discuss and decide if you wish to alter any of your reflective key words or phrases. What have you learned through this process?

> *For me, this skill is a reminder that while I may not have control over some of the situations I have confronted, I do have the power to change my perspective (fig. 4–4).*

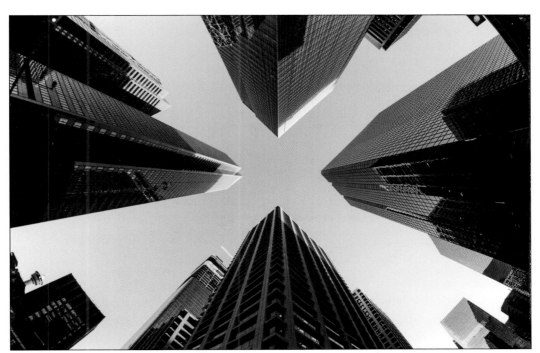

Fig. 4–4. What is your perspective? (unsplash.com)

NOTES

1   Reivich, Karen and Andrew Shatté. *The Resiliency Factor: 7 Keys to Finding Your Inner Strength and Overcoming Life's Hurdles*. New York: Broadway Books, 2002, 168-185.

2   Pattakos, Alex and Elaine Dundon. *Prisoners of Our Thoughts: Viktor Frankl's Principles for Discovering Meaning in Life and Work*. Oakland, CA: Berrett-Koehler Publishers, 2017.

3   Bridges, William and Susan Bridges. *Managing Transitions: Making the Most of Change*. Boston: Da Capo Press, 2017.

4   American Psychological Association. "10 Tips for Building Resilience in Children and Teens." http://www. apa.org/helpcenter/resilience.aspx.

5   Colman, Andrew M. *A Dictionary of Psychology*. New York: Oxford University Press, 2015.

6   Mayer, John D., David R. Caruso, and Peter Salovey. "Emotional intelligence meets traditional standards for an intelligence." *Intelligence* 27, no. 4 (1999): 267-298.

7   Goleman, Daniel. *Emotional Intelligence: Why It Can Matter More than IQ*. New York: Bantam Books, 2005.

8   Bar-On, Reuven and James D. A. Parker, eds. *The Handbook of Emotional Intelligence: Theory, Development, Assessment, and Application at Home, School, and in the Workplace*. San Francisco: Jossey-Bass Inc., 2000.

9   Bennis, Warren. "Become a Tomorrow Leader." In Spears, Larry C. and Michele Lawrence, eds. *Focus on Leadership: Servant-Leadership for the 21st Century*. New York: John Wiley & Sons, 2002, 101-109.

10   Bennis, Warren. "Why Servant-Leadership Matters." In Spears, Larry C. and Michele Lawrence, eds. *Practicing Servant-Leadership: Succeeding through Trust, Bravery, and Forgiveness*. San Francisco: Josey-Bass, 2004.

11   Sinek, Simon. "Why Leaders Eat Last." https://www.youtube.com/watch?v=ReRcHdeUG9Y.

12   Bennis, Warren G. and Robert J. Thomas. "Crucibles of leadership." *Harvard Business Review* 80, no. 9 (2002): 39-43, 124.

13   Thomas, Robert J. and Peter Cheese. "Leadership: Experience is the best teacher." *Strategy & Leadership* 33, no. 3 (2005): 24-29.

14   Calhoun, Lawrence G. and Richard G. Tedeschi. *Handbook of Posttraumatic Growth: Research and Practice*. New York: Routledge, 2014.

15   Barskova, Tatjana and Rainer Oesterreich. "Post-traumatic growth in people living with a serious medical condition and its relations to physical and mental health: A systematic review." *Disability and Rehabilitation* 31, no. 21 (2009): 1709-1733.

16   Sledge, William H., James A. Boydstun, and Alton J. Rabe. "Self-concept changes related to war captivity." *Archives of General Psychiatry* 37, no. 4 (1980): 430-44.

17   Marien, Hans, Henk Aarts, and Ruud Custers. "Being flexible or rigid in goal-directed behavior: When positive affect implicitly motivates the pursuit of goals or means." *Journal of Experimental Social Psychology* 48, no. 1 (2012): 277-283.

18   Meiran, Nachshon. "Task switching: Mechanisms underlying rigid vs. flexible self-control." In Hassin, Ran R., Kevin N. Ochsner, and Yaacov Trope, eds. *Self Control in Society, Mind, and Brain*. New York: Oxford University Press, 2010, 202-220.

19   Tugade, Michele M., Barbara L. Fredrickson, and Lisa Feldman Barrett. "Psychological resilience and positive emotional granularity: Examining the benefits of positive emotions on coping and health." *Journal of Personality* 72, no. 6 (2004): 1161-1190.

20   Kashdan, Todd B. and Jonathan Rottenberg. "Psychological flexibility as a fundamental aspect of health." *Clinical Psychology Review* 30, no. 7 (2010): 865-878.

21   Crum, Alia J., Modupe Akinola, Ashley Martin, and Sean Fath. "The role of stress mindset in shaping cognitive, emotional, and physiological responses to challenging and threatening stress." *Anxiety, Stress, & Coping* 30, no. 4 (2017): 379-395.

22   Fisher, P. Brian. "Resilience thinking in higher education: Institutional resilience as a sustainability goal." In Filho, Walter L., Mark Mifsud, Chris Shiel, and Rudi Pretorius, eds. *Handbook of Theory and Practice of Sustainable Development in Higher Education* vol. 3. Cham: Springer International Publishing, 2017, 209-222.

23   Chrysani, Athina, Panagiotis Kalogerakis, and Athanassios Katsis. "The road to resilience: Breaking the cycle of disadvantage." *Educational Journal of the University of Patras UNESCO Chair* 4, no. 1 (2017): 71-82.

24   Bandura, Albert. "Social cognitive theory: An agentic perspective." *Asian Journal of Social Psychology*, 2, no. 1 (1999): 21-41.

25   Fredrickson, Barbara L., Michele M. Tugade, Christian E. Waugh, and Gregory R. Larkin. "What good are positive emotions in crises? A prospective study of resilience and emotions following the terrorist attacks on the United States on September 11th, 2001." *Journal of Personality and Social Psychology* 84 no. 2 (2003): 365-376.

26   Tedeschi, Richard G. and Lawrence G. Calhoun. "The posttraumatic growth inventory: Measuring the positive legacy of trauma." *Journal of Traumatic Stress* 9 no. 3 (1996): 455-471.

27   Joseph, Stephen. "Growth following adversity: Positive psychological perspectives on posttraumatic stress." *Psychological Topics* 18 no. 2 (2009): 335-344.

28   Tedeschi, Richard G. and Lawrence G. Calhoun. "A clinical approach to posttraumatic growth." In Linley, P. Alex and Stephen Joseph, eds. *Positive Psychology in Practice*. Hoboken, New Jersey: Wiley & Sons, Inc., 2004, 405-419.

29   Bennett, Mary P., Janice M. Zeller, Lisa Rosenberg, and Judith McCann. "The effect of mirthful laughter on stress and natural killer cell activity." *Alternative Therapies in Health and Medicine* 9, no. 2 (2003): 38-45.

30   Christie, Wanda and Carol Moore. "The impact of humor on patients with cancer." *Clinical Journal of Oncology Nursing* 9 no. 2 (2005): 211-218.

31   Futterman, A. D., M. E. Kemeny, D. Shapiro, and J. L. Fahey. "Immunological and physiological changes associated with induced positive and negative mood." *Psychosomatic Medicine* 56 no. 6 (1994): 499–511.

32   Fry, William F. "The biology of humor." *Humor: International Journal of Humor Research* 7, no. 2 (1994): 111-126.

33   LaRouche, Loretta. *Relax—You May Only Have a Few Minutes Left: Using the Power of Humor to Overcome Stress in Your Life and Work*. New York: Villard, 1998, 21-25.

34   Martin, Rod A. and Herbert M. Lefcourt. "Sense of humor as a moderator of the relation between stressors and moods." *Journal of Personality and Social Psychology* 45, no. 6 (1983): 1313-1324.

35   Weisenberg, Matisyohu, Inbal Tepper, and Joseph Schwarzwald. "Humor as a cognitive technique for increasing pain tolerance." *Pain* 63 no. 2 (1995): 207-212.

36   Shantinath, S. D. "What if we brushed our minds like we brushed our teeth?" *Azcentral.com*, February 2, 2014. http://www.azcentral.com/opinions/articles/20140202preventive-mental-health-care-floss-shantinath-viewpoints.html.

37   İşmen, A. Esra. "Emotional intelligence and problem solving." *Marmara Üniversitesi Egitim Bilimleri Dergisi* 13, no. 13 (2011): 111-124.

38   Jordan, Peter J. and Ashlea C. Troth. "Managing emotions during team problem solving: Emotional intelligence and conflict resolution." *Human Performance* 17, no. 2 (2004): 195-218.

39   Kerrigan, Deanna, Kelly Johnson, Miriam Stewart, Trish Magyari, Nancy Hutton, Jonathan M. Ellen, and Erica M. S. Sibinga. "Perceptions, experiences, and shifts in perspective occurring among urban youth participating in a mindfulness-based stress reduction program." *Complementary Therapies in Clinical Practice* 17, no. 2 (2011): 96-101.

40   Bates, Timothy C. and Shivani Gupta. "Smart groups of smart people: Evidence for IQ as the origin of collective intelligence in the performance of human groups." *Intelligence* 60, no. 1 (2017): 46-56.

41   Kopcha, Theodore J. "A systems-based approach to technology integration using mentoring and communities of practice." *Educational Technology Research and Development* 58, no. 2 (2010): 175-190.

5

BELIEF BUILDING

Every thought is a seed. If you plant crab apples,
don't count on harvesting Golden Delicious.

— Bill Meyer

OVERVIEW

Why: Thoughts and beliefs drive our feelings and behaviors. The good news is our thoughts and beliefs are modifiable. Identifying and modifying self-defeating thoughts or beliefs, those that bring about undesirable consequences, can lower our stress.

How: There are a number of ways that we can examine and change those beliefs and attitudes that increase our stress. The ABC approach considers adversity or activating event (A), beliefs or thoughts (B), and consequences or feelings and behaviors (C). Recognizing that all beliefs bring about consequences permits adjustment to bring about appropriate change. The steps of ABC look like this:

- Identify the activating event, belief, and consequence.

- Assess the value of the belief.

- Identify any self-defeating thoughts and more realistic beliefs.

- Establish a goal-setting process to bring about any appropriate change.

Other skills include increasing our emotional intelligence, practicing positivity, developing a more flexible mind-set, and practicing gratitude. Focusing on those things we have control over rather than things beyond our control can help us cope with stress more effectively and actually increase our self-efficacy.[1,2]

> *The world we have created is a product of our thinking;*
> *it cannot be changed without changing our thinking.*

— Albert Einstein

Identifying a measure of change between before and after developing the goal and steps to meet the goal provides us a measure of our success. We use the Subjective Units of Distress Scale (SUDS) to help subjectively identify stress levels before, and again after, as somewhere between zero (0) and ten (10), where 0 corresponds to no stress and 10 to the highest level of stress you have ever experienced. The anticipation is that the SUDS level begins to decrease even after developing a goal statement and defining the steps to attain the goal. If the SUDS level increases, then take some time to reassess the goal statement to assure it is attainable.

And reassess the steps to assure that they have been adequately defined and there are a sufficient number. After all, you want to be able to check off each step and mark progress toward reaching your goal.

Goal Setting Skill—Belief Building

The way we view the world creates and reinforces our world view. But does this view help or hurt? Maybe some views work and some don't.

Rate the stress level you perceive

Analog SUDS	Digital SUDS	Emoji SUDS
Actually, I'm not stressed	0	
A little stressed	1–3	
Somewhat stressed	4–6	
Quite a bit stressed	7–8	
It's really bad	9	
Run and hide!!	10	

Think about what's stressing you out. What might help?

Recognize the activating event (A).

Review any expected consequences (C).

What perceived beliefs (B) led you there?

Try and identify an objective to help you do these.

Now it's time to figure out how to get there.

Write out your belief goal statement and how you plan to get there, step-by-step.

Use the systems below as suggested approaches.

Now get started! Don't be shy. Go for it!

Have you made any progress?

Rate the stress level you perceive now

Is it lower?

Yes	No
Congratulations!! You did it!! Now you can do this whenever you need it!	What might have gone wrong? Did you figure out all your steps? Did you actually do them all? Did you give yourself enough time? Give it another try, from the beginning.

Breaking all this down

An activating event (A) can be anything, including just contemplating challenging our beliefs. However, more often the (A) will be some external event (e.g., an important final exam, a call to return to a domestic violence scene, or a field call to your emergency department saying multiple injuries are on their way to your hospital).

Whatever the activating event might be, it will precipitate our perceived consequences (C), which are typically our feelings. Do these feelings help us mobilize our resources or do they become an obstacle for us being able to perform at our peak?

Here's the clincher: What is the belief (B) that brought you here? Maybe you are straining under some self-defeating thoughts that are increasing your stress? Keep in mind that, with the ABCs identified, you can re-examine any of your self-defeating thoughts and/or beliefs and identify a more realistic belief. I know this is hard, but you know you can do it! And, when you've got it, consider adopting or sustaining this new belief.

Is SUDS the only option for measuring change? Certainly not! You are encouraged to find the most appropriate measurement for your needs. The only thing that matters is that it can provide meaningful feedback with regard to change, or even transformation, resulting from applying the goal-setting process. Perhaps a scale that measures the likelihood of completing the task might be more useful. That scale might range from 0 to 10, where 0 corresponds to no chance of completion and 10 is fully sure of completion. If you were using a likelihood-of-completion scale, then you would anticipate an increase in likelihood to complete from premeasure to postmeasure.

> *In order to carry a positive action, we must develop here a positive vision.*
>
> — Dalai Lama

WHY BELIEF BUILDING?

We all have patterns, beliefs, or ways of thinking that are comfortable, but these can also be destructive. Our thoughts drive our behavior. These thoughts, however, are modifiable. We can affect the way in which we think. Self-defeating patterns of thinking have negative consequences for us (fig. 5–1). They will impact our relationships and our ability to enjoy life.

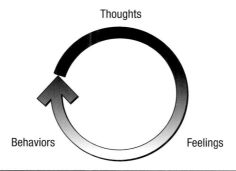

Fig. 5–1. Cycle of self-defeating thought patterns

Unfortunately, there is considerable evidence that, as human beings, we tend to be more negative than positive in our thinking.[3,4,5] From an evolutionary perspective, this makes sense.

Millennia ago, when we'd walk out of our cave in the morning, our first thoughts were probably not about the beautiful sunrise. Instead, we would be focused on looking around to make sure some saber-toothed tiger wasn't going to have us for breakfast. While this kind of thinking may have been of value to us in the past, today its effects can be detrimental to our well-being, both personally and professionally. This is not to say that there are not times when negative thinking can be appropriate and necessary.[6,7] Unfortunately, we tend to be biased toward negative thinking and actually consider those who offer us negative feedback as smarter than those who offer more positive input.[8] Interestingly, it can be detrimental to try and change a negative thinker's way of processing information, since telling someone to think positively can backfire and make the person think even more negatively.[9] It is when such thinking patterns become habits that we can run into problems, especially in how we view ourselves, other people, and the world.[10,11,12] Such negative thinking habits can then impact our relationships with those we love and care about.[13]

You can't stop the waves, but you can learn how to surf.

—Jon Kabat-Zinn

THE HOW OF BUILDING BELIEFS

There are multitudes of ways that we can confront our negative thinking. One way is to explore our mind-set. There are basically two kinds of mind-sets: a flexible, or growth, mind-set and the fixed, or rigid, mind-set.[14] A growth mind-set is based on our belief that our basic qualities can be developed through our efforts. While we may differ in our abilities and aptitudes, interests, or temperaments, those of us with a growth mind-set believe everyone can change and grow through practice and experience.[15,16] Those with a fixed mind-set believe that whatever traits, intelligence, and abilities they or others have is fixed and unlikely to change. Such outlooks can have profound ramifications on the quality of our lives.

This is especially true in education where students with flexible mind-sets are more likely to be successful.[17,18,19,20,21] Even within the first responder community, mind-set can play an important role in one's ability to cope with the challenges of the work.[22,23,24] With the ever-increasing demands within the nursing profession, a flexible mind-set is imperative to long-term career survival.[25,26,27] In addition, by understanding our emotional intelligence we can also create a more flexible mind-set.[28]

While self-defeating thought patterns can have a negative impact on our lives, the good news is that we can learn to change what and how we think. But we must first understand and identify our thoughts and how they impact our moods.

Too often, we berate ourselves for not being good enough, thinking about how we or others should or should not have done something, and using what has been referred to as a *shouldarrhea* mind-set. Perhaps we spend too much of our time thinking about our flaws, foibles, and mess-ups. Or, we measure ourselves against some unrealistic ideal, such as a character from a movie or TV show, and we inevitably come up short. What impact do these thoughts have on our mood? They can be self-defeating and certainly do not help us to attain realistic goals. Further, these self-defeating thought patterns can lead to some rather negative consequences such as depression, anxiety, poor self-esteem, anger at others, isolation, and poor performance in work and relationships. These, in due course, impact our general physical health, mental health, and social well-being.

Having the courage to identify and confront our self-defeating thoughts is another way to improve our beliefs about ourselves, our abilities, and our beliefs about others.[29]

David Burns observed the following self-defeating thoughts:[30]

- **All-or-nothing thinking.** This can be summed up as thinking in terms of black and white or absolutes. If we don't do things perfectly, then we see ourselves as complete failures. We tend to see one mistake as a total disaster. When caught in this line of thinking, we focus only on the mistakes that we made, rather than acknowledging the good that we did and the ways in which we contributed positively to the lives of others. For example, there is, unfortunately, the mind-set within an emergency medical services organization that "one mistake can screw up a thousand attaboys." Paramedics may focus only on the very few people they lost and lose sight of the many lives they saved.

- **Overgeneralization.** This happens when the evaluation of an isolated event or behavior on the part of some individual is misconstrued as a general conclusion. When we overgeneralize, we tend to see a single negative outcome as the beginning of a never-ending pattern of defeat. Words that indicate that we are using this self-defeating thought are "always" and "never." For example, getting in an argument with your partner and saying "You never listen to me" or "We always have to do everything your way." Another example of overgeneralization would be if John Smith asks you a dumb question and suddenly all Smiths are idiots. We can even limit the scope of our social relationships by buying into stereotypes or making hasty generalizations about other people.

- **Mental filter.** This involves focusing on a single, usually negative, detail to the exclusion of all else. We focus only on that which confirms our biases and overlook conflicting evidence. If we view the world as an unsafe place where no one is to be trusted, we may then look for people and situations that confirm our belief and ignore or discount situations and people that are not consistent with this view.

- **Discounting the positive.** When complimented for a job well done, we respond with something akin to, "I was just doing my job." We focus on what we could have done better and talk about ways that we could improve rather than acknowledging what we have done well. While continuous improvement is a worthy goal, we all need to take time to smell the roses and enjoy our successes. A dark side of this type of thinking is that others quit complimenting us because we discount their compliments. This kind of thinking takes the joy out of life and can lead to a sense of inadequacy. For example, consider an annual performance evaluation process where the individual being evaluated focuses on a single negative element with the belief that this is proof of an overall subpar performance, despite receiving an above average rating for the year. How many of us have trouble taking a compliment? How many of us discount positive feedback by saying, "I was just doing my job"?

- **Jumping to conclusions.** When we jump to conclusions, we typically make a negative interpretation of a situation or person with little or no supporting evidence. Variations of this include mind reading and fortune-telling:

  - **Mind reading** occurs when we assume that someone is reacting to us negatively (or even positively) without any evidence to support such a conclusion. For example, you enter a house and observe a family member who seems to be scowling at you. You think, "that person sure looks angry." You subsequently learn, however, that the person suffered a stroke several years ago, resulting in paralysis of some facial muscles.

– **Fortune-telling** is another form of this cognitive distortion in which we predict negative (or even positive) outcomes without supporting evidence. Such jumping to conclusions may lead to negative, self-fulfilling prophecies such that when we predict a negative outcome we unconsciously act in ways that ensure that negative outcome is realized. For example, consider the outcome if individuals with PTSD conclude they will be messed up for the rest of their lives.

– **Magnification and minimization.** This typically occurs when we unreasonably exaggerate the importance of one set of characteristics or evidence, usually negative, and minimize the importance of another set of characteristics or evidence, usually positive. Catastrophizing or, alternatively, minimizing the significance of an event, can cloud our ability to put things into perspective. For example, we exaggerate our flaws, foibles, and failures and minimize the importance of our positive characteristics such as empathy, the value of service, the understanding of self-sacrifice, and the ability to survive in adverse circumstances. This can, and perhaps should, be referred to as the *binocular trick*.

– **Emotional reasoning.** Here we use our personal or subjective emotions as evidence of an actual or objective reality. This can be especially problematic for individuals who see themselves as particularly intuitive, whereby they may begin to believe that they have developed their intuition to the point where they can predict the future based on a feeling. "I feel anxious, therefore something bad is going to happen" can be problematic for individuals who have developed and honed their vigilance skills, as they begin to believe that they can intuit or predict the future. Recognize that all of us have learned to pick up cues in our environments that permit us to anticipate possible and even probable future events. However, this is not through our feelings or emotions. An example might be the emotional fallout from the 9/11 event whereby some people had feelings of anger and fear toward people of Middle Eastern heritage and came to believe that all people of Middle Eastern heritage pose a threat.

– **Should statements.** These are frequently called *parental injunctions* and often incorporate words such as should, shouldn't, have to, ought to, or must. We focus on *should have done* or *shouldn't have done*, rather than on actual events. For example, a paramedic may return from a difficult pediatric call unable to stop hammering himself or herself with the idea that "I should have been able to get that intubation." Trauma survivors can experience what is called a "hypersense of justice," a combination of all-or-nothing thinking and should statements. This type of thinking applies yet another set of rigid internal rules that can lead to guilt and apathy—not the motivation needed to face complex problems with mental clarity and resolve.

There are a couple of catchphrases that remind us of the destruction of these types of statements, like "Don't should all over yourself" and "Stop should-ing on yourself." In fact, here is an interesting exercise to monitor your use of these statements. Take a 3×5 card and for a 24-hour period, put a check mark on it every time you say or think the words should, shouldn't, have to, ought to, or must: "I have to get my homework done." "I should have worked harder to save that patient."

"I shouldn't be impacted by the traumas I see." "I must get my act together." It will surprise most of us to see how often we engage in this kind of destructive talk. Now add to that all of the times we think about others and how they should and shouldn't behave. You'd better get another 3×5 card! The point is that such thinking only increases our stress and decreases our self-efficacy. Consider using the word *want* rather than *should*, as in "I want to get my act together."

- **Labeling and mislabeling.** Burns notes that labeling is an extreme form of all-or-nothing thinking. Instead of considering the subtlety and complexity of a situation or behavior, we apply a label to it and consider it an unalterable fact. For example, a student who fails an exam after neglecting to adequately study may self-label as "stupid" and consider this state as unalterable. This is self-defeating, as it leaves no room for improving the poor study habits. Labeling and mislabeling may use abstractions as fact, such as describing people as fools, idiots, or jerks. This mind-set drastically limits our ability to act constructively toward other people. This applies not only to people but to other things as well. Think of the last time you were in a traffic jam and thought, "I'll never take this road again!"

- **Personalization and blame.** We assign personal responsibility where the target of our blame, be it ourselves or others, has little or no control over the situation or outcome. Whether it is directed at ourselves or others, this mind-set creates the perception that we have far more power than is actually the case. If we use this kind of thinking during a crisis, we neglect critical relevant information such as, "Did I have control over the people who sent me here?" "Did I have control over what other individuals decided to do?" "Did I have control over what caused the crisis?" Personalization of this type leads to guilt and shame.

  Blame occurs when we unilaterally assign responsibility to others for the situation. For example, "My marriage sucks because my husband works a 24-hour shift and is never home," or "The reason I drink is because of the people I deal with on a daily basis." These are not effective ways of dealing with problems because they can lead to irrational guilt or shame, as well as feelings of apathy or anger.

Researchers have observed other patterns of self-defeating thoughts.[31,32] Those with PTSD or anxiety disorders are particularly prone to what are termed *avoidant thoughts*.[33,34] These thoughts cause us to engage in safety behaviors such as avoidance and even trying to escape. Examples of these types of thoughts include "Crowds make me nervous, so I'll just stay home" or "I'm not good at tests, so I'll just call in sick." These thoughts prevent us from fully living our lives and serve only to reinforce our fears and anxieties (fig. 5–2).

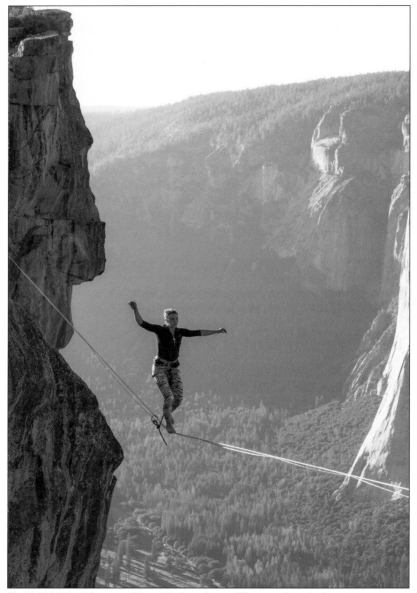

Fig. 5–2. Maintaining a positive attitude makes a difference. (unsplash.com)

A positive attitude may not solve all your problems,
but it will annoy enough people to make it worth the effort.

—Herm Albright

Example:

Baseline SUDS (0–10)

    Activating event (situation)

        Belief (I think…)

            Consequence (I feel…)

SUDS intensity SUDS = 5

> Activating event   Seeing a driver speeding through heavy traffic.
>
> Belief   Questions the sanity and ability of the speeding driver.
>
> Consequence   Became angered and verbally lashed out at the speeding driver.

Now it's time to put all this to work:

- Identify self-defeating thoughts.
- Form a more realistic view of the situation.
- Examine any resultant change of feelings.
- Evaluate any change in your SUDS (0–10).

> Self-defeating thoughts: May have been jumping to a conclusion that did not correctly describe the situation.
>
> Realistic view: Maybe the person was speeding to the hospital and was going there to address the need of a family member.
>
> Change of view: Realized that there may be more to the situation than at first perceived.

SUDS intensity SUDS = 1

> *The only difference between a good day and a bad day is your attitude.*
>
> — Dennis S. Brown

GRATITUDE

Another tool to build a healthier belief system is to practice gratitude (fig. 5–3). Practicing gratitude can have not only an effect on our outlook on life, but also a positive impact on our overall health as well.[35,36,37] Those who practice gratitude are able to cope better with life stresses and have a greater belief in themselves and their abilities.[38,39]

Consider this exercise, which can be done at night as you lie in bed. Think of five things you are grateful for. Be creative. Consider people, places, things. And don't forget your pets! Then really focus on each one and reflect in as much detail as you can about them. When you think about them, how do you feel about yourself and your life? What is your SUDS as you think about these things you are grateful for? Now what would your SUDS likely be if you were to focus on things that you needed to get done tomorrow, or engaged in a critical review of what you didn't accomplish during the day? If you want to reduce your stress, pick the things you are grateful for.

> *Gratitude is the sign of noble souls.*
>
> — Aesop

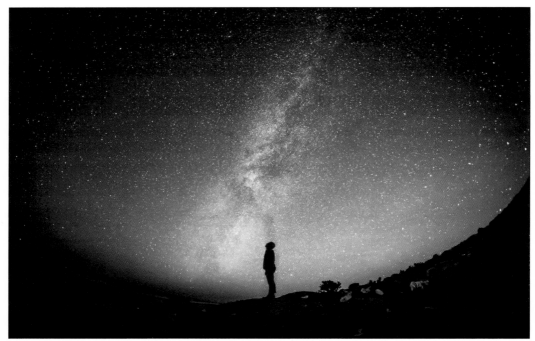

Fig. 5–3. What are you grateful for? (unsplash.com)

INTERNALIZE BELIEF BUILDING

Recall, in as much detail as possible, a past personal experience where you practiced *belief building*. That is, an instance where you consciously thought about what your belief was at the time and what consequences you were addressing; perhaps you had fallen into a self-defeating thought. Given your exposure to belief building, translate it into a belief-building skill. If you prefer, consider writing about your experience as a short story as a way to exercise the belief-building skill. And don't be shy! The more details you can remember, the more likely you are to feel empowered to use this skill in the future. You can work on this process individually or in collaboration.

- Consider a past personal situation where you successfully used belief building.
- Establish, as best you recall, your baseline SUDS (0–10).
- Identify, as best you recall, the activating event, the belief it raised, and what was the resulting consequence.
- Assess the value of that belief.
- Identify any self-defeating thoughts.
- Focus on what more realistic beliefs you might consider.
- Assess, as best you can recall, what your SUDS level (0–10) became after applying the skill and considering the consequences.
- Identify any other skills you used in this exercise.
- Assess whether obtaining the SUDS, identifying the stressors and fears, and identifying alternatives might have made the process more manageable and compelling.

- Identify changes, if any, you might make to the skill to make it more personally useful.
- Assess your personal confidence in being ready and able to apply this skill to meet any future needs.

As you think about this past event and your ability to develop a more realistic belief, what thoughts and feelings come to mind? You can also use the following form to record your responses.

ABC worksheet

Activating event (the challenge)

Belief (I think…)

Consequence (I feel/I do…)

SUDS intensity (0–10)   SUDS = _____

What self-defeating thoughts are being used?

_____

What is a more realistic way of thinking about this situation?

_____

How does this more realistic view change your feelings?

_____

Be aware of your thoughts; they become words.
Be aware of your words; they become actions.
Be aware of your actions; they become habits.
Be aware of your habits; they become character.
Be aware of your character; it becomes destiny.

— Chinese proverb

EXTERNALIZE: APPLY BELIEF BUILDING AS A GROUP

Using the ABC worksheet, you have reflected on how you have used the skill of belief building in your own life. Given these tools, examine the following case study.

Case study: You are the charge nurse assisting with the care of a five-year-old boy who has been kicked in the stomach repeatedly by an abusive father. You notice that one of the techs is visibly upset and near tears. After a private discussion, the tech admits to having some difficulty dealing with this situation because of the five-year-old in the tech's own family. The tech expresses a feeling of helplessness in this situation and that there is more that should be done.

Reflect: This is a tough case study, even to write about. However, for those is the healthcare field it will be an all-too-frequent reality and you need the skills to help yourself and others cope with these harsh facts of life (fig. 5–4). Using TAPPS, collaborative groups will develop a possible intervention to the case study. Remember that you can use all of the skills we have explored up to this point to help this young tech.

ABC worksheet

    Activating event (the challenge)

        Belief (I think…)

            Consequence (I feel/I do…)

SUDS intensity (0–10)   SUDS = _____

    What self-defeating thoughts are being used?

_____

    What is a more realistic way of thinking about this situation?

_____

    How does this more realistic view change the feelings?

_____

We cannot direct the wind but we can adjust the sails.

— Author unknown

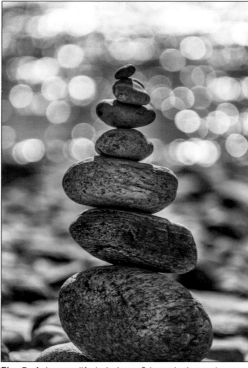

Fig. 5–4. Is your life in balance? (unsplash.com)

PRACTICE BELIEF BUILDING

Again, one of the best ways we can really integrate a skill into our lives is to make it personal. To do this, we need to see the value of it in our lives. Thinking about and applying the belief-building skill in our lives makes it more likely that we will remember the skill. Therefore, consider how you would best incorporate the concept of belief building into your current life. While the ABC approach can be an effective method for determining self-defeating thoughts or beliefs that bring about undesirable consequences, ABC can also be used to identify robust beliefs that subsequently bring about very desirable consequences. Specifically, consider applying belief building to a current adversity you are facing. Alternatively, consider a past situation where you experienced or witnessed a very positive consequence following some activating event. Then, try to identify the B-C connection.

ABC worksheet

Activating event (the challenge)

Belief (I think...)

Consequence (I feel/I do...)

SUDS intensity (0–10)   SUDS = _____

What self-defeating thoughts are being used?

_____

What is a more realistic way of thinking about this situation?

_____

How does this more realistic view change the feelings?

_____

Another cognitive diffusion skill is to first allow yourself to bring to mind a disturbing and negative self-judgment that takes the form of "I am X," such as "I am a failure" or "I am inadequate."[40,41] Allow yourself to hold that thought for several seconds and place some belief in the thought. Notice what happens.

Reflect: How does maintaining that thought affect you?

_____
_____
_____
_____

Next, allow yourself to take the thought "I am X," but insert the phrase "I am having *the thought* that...." As before, allow yourself to hold that thought for several seconds and place some belief in the thought, but this time with the new phrase. Notice what happens.

_____

_____

_____

_____

Reflect: How does maintaining that thought affect you? At the end of this simple exercise, most of us feel more distant from the disturbing thought and it thus has less impact on our overall feelings.

_____

_____

_____

_____

Reflect: Does identifying your ABCs make you more aware of the beliefs you are maintaining? Do these beliefs lead to either desirable or undesirable consequences for you?

_____

_____

_____

_____

Most people think that their only option is to change their circumstances.
But these are not the true cause of their unhappiness.
It has more to do with the way they think about their circumstances.

— David Michie

APPLY BELIEF BUILDING TO YOUR COMMUNITY

Community can be defined as any group of people living, working, or sharing common interests, such as a family, team, work group, or neighborhood. You have applied the belief-building skill to yourself and to another person as a small group exercise. Is this a prevailing self-defeating belief within your community that the community could benefit from examining using this exercise? What are the implications of expanding this skill to a community of individuals?

Consider a community situation where you might use the belief-building skill.

Checklist for Applying Belief Building to Your Community

Baseline SUDS (0–10)

    Activating event (the challenge)

        Belief (I think…)

            Consequence (I feel/I do…)

Baseline SUDS	SUDS = ?
Consider:	What is the value of our beliefs as they are now?
	How do you think this event will play out and conclude?
	What changes, if any, might you make to the skill to make it more useful?
	How does this more realistic view change the feelings?
Follow-up SUDS	SUDS = ?
	Do you feel comfortable and ready to become a mentor?
	How confident do you feel in applying this skill to meet the needs?

One obvious place we can apply this skill is within our families. Practicing the power of affirmations to our children and partners can have a positive impact on those we care for the most.[42,43,44] Working on creating and modeling a flexible mind-set can help create a more resilient family.[45,46,47]

> *Once you replace negative thoughts with positive ones,*
> *you'll start having positive results.*
>
> — Willie Nelson

REMEMBERING BELIEF BUILDING

We have examined and applied the belief-building skill. Take the opportunity now to reflect on the skill and associate some key words or phrases that help to succinctly define the skill using your own words. When you have completed this process, compare these key words and phrases with the person or persons with whom you are working. Discuss and decide if you wish to alter any of your reflective key words or phrases. What have you learned through this process?

_____

_____

_____

_____

> *All action results from thought, so it is thoughts that matter.*
>
> — Sai Baba

NOTES

1   Bandura, Albert. *Self-efficacy: The Exercise of Control*. New York: Macmillan, 1997.

2   Bandura, Albert. "Self-efficacy mechanism in human agency." *American Psychologist* 37, no. 2 (1982): 122-147.

3   Kertz, Sarah J., Kimberly T. Stevens, and Keith P. Klein. "The association between attention control, anxiety, and depression: The indirect effects of repetitive negative thinking and mood recovery." *Anxiety, Stress, & Coping* 30, no. 4 (2016): 1-13.

4   Williams, Megan. "Book review. Breaking negative thinking patterns: A schema therapy self-help and support book." *Behavioural and Cognitive Psychotherapy* 44, no. 4 (2016): 510-511.

5   Greenberg, Melanie. *The Stress-Proof Brain: Master Your Emotional Response to Stress Using Mindfulness and Neuroplasticity*. Oakland, CA: New Harbinger Publications, 2017.

6   Couzin-Frankel, Jennifer. "The power of negative thinking." *Science* 342, no. 6154 (2013): 68-69.

7   Norem, Julie. *The Positive Power of Negative Thinking: Using 'Defensive Pessimism' to Manage Anxiety and Perform at Your Peak*. Cambridge, MA: Basic Books, 2001.

8   Nass, Clifford and Corina Yen. *The Man Who Lied to His Laptop: What We Can Learn about Ourselves from Our Machines*. New York: Penguin, 2010.

9   Henion, Andy and Jason Moser. "Positive, negative thinkers' brains revealed." *MSUToday*. http://msutoday. msu.edu/news/2014/positive-negative-thinkers-brains-revealed/.

10 Verplanken, Bas, Oddgeir Friborg, Catharina E. Wang, David Trafimow, and Kristin Woolf. "Mental habits: Metacognitive reflection on negative self-thinking." *Journal of Personality and Social Psychology* 92, no. 3 (2007): 526-541.

11 Schwartz, Jeffrey M. and Rebecca Gladding. *You Are Not Your Brain: The 4-Step Solution for Changing Bad Habits, Ending Unhealthy Thinking, and Taking Control of Your Life*. New York: Penguin, 2011.

12 Paul, Richard W. and Linda Elder. *Critical Thinking: Tools for Taking Charge of Your Professional and Personal Life*. Upper Saddle River, NJ: Pearson Education, 2013.

13 Fincham, Frank D. and Thomas N. Bradbury. "The impact of attributions in marriage: A longitudinal analysis." *Journal of Personality and Social Psychology* 53, no. 3 (1987): 510-517.

14 Dweck, Carol S. *Mindset: The New Psychology of Success*. New York: Random House Digital, Inc., 2008.

15 Dweck, Carol S. *Mindset-Updated Edition: Changing the Way You Think to Fulfil Your Potential*. London: Robinson, 2017.

16 Kastner, Justin, Alyson Lister, Antoinette Cutler, and McNeil Dolliver. "Leveraging insights from psychology for pedagogical innovation." *Honors in Higher Education* 1, no. 1 (2016).

17 Yeager, David S., Carissa Romero, Dave Paunesku, Christopher S. Hulleman, Barbara Schneider, Cintia Hinojosa, Hae Yeon Lee, et al. "Using design thinking to improve psychological interventions: The case of the growth mindset during the transition to high school." *Journal of Educational Psychology* 108, no. 3 (2016): 374-391.

18 Lyubomirsky, Sonja and Susan Nolen-Hoeksema. "Effects of self-focused rumination on negative thinking and interpersonal problem solving." *Journal of Personality and Social Psychology* 69, no. 1 (1995): 176-190.

19 Schroder, Hans S., Matthew M. Yalch, Sindes Dawood, Courtney P. Callahan, M. Brent Donnellan, and Jason S. Moser. "Growth mindset of anxiety buffers the link between stressful life events and psychological distress and coping strategies." *Personality and Individual Differences* 110 (2017): 23-26.

20 Yeager, David Scott and Carol S. Dweck. "Mindsets that promote resilience: When students believe that personal characteristics can be developed." *Educational Psychologist* 47, no. 4 (2012): 302-314.

21 Morrison, Gale M. and Megan Redding Allen. "Promoting student resilience in school contexts." *Theory into Practice* 46, no. 2 (2007): 162-169.

22 Dowdall-Thomae, Cynthia, John Gilkey, Wanda Larson, and Rebecca Arend-Hicks. "Elite firefighter/first responder mindsets and outcome coping efficacy." *International Journal of Emergency Mental Health* 14, no. 4 (2012): 269-281.

23 Deppa, Karen F. et al. "Major factors that influence behavioral health in the fire service." In Deppa, Karen F. and Judith Saltzberg. *Resilience Training for Firefighters: An Approach to Prevent Behavioral Health Problems*. Cham: Springer International Publishing, 2016, 35-50.

24 Russell, Eric J. "Serving the responders growth." In *In Command of Guardians: Executive Servant Leadership for the Community of Responders*. Cham: Springer International Publishing, 2017, 73-87.

25 Doherty, Tanya M. and Minette Coetzee. "Community health workers and professional nurses: Defining the roles and understanding the relationships." *Public Health Nursing* 22, no. 4 (2005): 360-365.

26   Sherwood, Gwen. "Driving forces for quality and safety: Changing mindsets to improve health care." In Sherwood, Gwen and Jane Barnsteiner. *Quality and Safety in Nursing: A Competency Approach to Improving Outcomes.* Chichester, West Sussex: Wiley-Blackwell, 2012, 3-21.

27   Foster, Roxanne Melissa Pinuka. "The power of emotional intelligence for facilitating psychologically flexible thinking: A contextual perspective in decision making and workplace flourishing" [doctorial thesis]. Canberra: Australian National University, 2016.

28   Gazelle, Gail, Jane M. Liebschutz, and Helen Riess. "Physician burnout: Coaching a way out." *Journal of General Internal Medicine 30, no. 4* (2015): 508-513.

29   Hardy, J. and E. J. Oliver. "Self-talk, positive thinking, and thought stopping." In Eklund, Robert C. and Gershon Tenebaum, eds. *Encyclopedia of Sport and Exercise Psychology.* Thousand Oaks, CA: Sage, 2014.

30   Burns, David D. *The Feeling Good Handbook.* New York: Penguin, 1999, 3-61.

31   Baumeister, Roy F. and Steven J. Scher. "Self-defeating behavior patterns among normal individuals: Review and analysis of common self-destructive tendencies." *Psychological Bulletin* 104, no. 1 (1988): 3-22.

32   Hope, Debra A., James D. Herbert, and Cameron White. "Diagnostic subtype, avoidant personality disorder, and efficacy of cognitive—behavioral group therapy for social phobia." *Cognitive Therapy and Research* 19, no. 4 (1995): 399-417.

33   Coroiu, Adina, Annett Körner, Shaunna Burke, Sarkis Meterissian, and Catherine M. Sabiston. "Stress and posttraumatic growth among survivors of breast cancer: A test of curvilinear effects." *International Journal of Stress Management* 23, no. 1 (2015): 84-97.

34   Smith, Jeffery. "Avoidance patterns and mechanisms." In *Psychotherapy.* Cham: Springer International Publishing, 2017, 41-50.

35   Emmons, Robert A. and Cheryl A. Crumpler. "Gratitude as a human strength: Appraising the evidence." *Journal of Social and Clinical Psychology* 19, no. 1 (2000): 56-69.

36   Hill, Patrick L., Mathias Allemand, and Brent W. Roberts. "Examining the pathways between gratitude and self-rated physical health across adulthood." *Personality and Individual Differences* 54, no. 1 (2013): 92-96.

37   Otey-Scott, Stacie. "A lesson in gratitude: exploring the salutogenic relationship between gratitude and health" [doctorial dissertation]. Virginia Beach: Regent University, 2007.

38   Dwiwardani, Carissa, Peter C. Hill, Richard A. Bollinger, Lashley E. Marks, et al. "Virtues develop from a secure base: Attachment and resilience as predictors of humility, gratitude, and forgiveness." *Journal of Psychology and Theology* 42, no. 1 (2014): 83-90.

39   Epstein, Ronald and Fred Marshall. "Beyond resilience: Cultivating compassion and gratitude (P12)." *Journal of Pain and Symptom Management* 53, no. 2 (2017): 309-310.

40   Masuda, Akihiko, Steven C. Hayes, Casey F. Sackett, and Michael P. Twohig. "Cognitive defusion and self-relevant negative thoughts: Examining the impact of a ninety-year-old technique." *Behaviour Research and Therapy* 42, no. 4 (2004): 477-485.

41   Donald, James N., Paul W. B. Atkins, Philip D. Parker, Alison M. Christie, and Jiesi Guo. "Cognitive defusion predicts more approach and less avoidance coping with stress, independent of threat and self-efficacy appraisals." *Journal of Personality* 85, no. 5 (2017): 716-729.

42   Pauketat, Janet V. T., Wesley G. Moons, Jacqueline M. Chen, Diane M. Mackie, and David K. Sherman. "Self-affirmation and affective forecasting: Affirmation reduces the anticipated impact of negative events." *Motivation and Emotion* 40, no. 5 (2016): 750-759.

43   Sherman, David K., Debra P. Bunyan, J. David Creswell, and Lisa M. Jaremka. "Psychological vulnerability and stress: The effects of self-affirmation on sympathetic nervous system responses to naturalistic stressors." *Health Psychology* 28, no. 5 (2009): 554-562.

44   Szente, Judit. "Empowering young children for success in school and in life." *Early Childhood Education Journal* 34, no. 6 (2007): 449-453.

45   Ganong, Lawrence H. and Marilyn Coleman. "Introduction to the special section: Family resilience in multiple contexts." *Journal of Marriage and Family* 64, no. 2 (2002): 346-348.

46   Walsh, Froma. *Strengthening Family Resilience.* New York: Guilford Publications, 2015.

47   Simon, Joan B., John J. Murphy, and Shelia M. Smith. "Understanding and fostering family resilience." *Family Journal* 13, no. 4 (2005): 427-436.

6

THRIVING

Surviving is important, but thriving is elegant.

— Maya Angelou

OVERVIEW

Why: Reflecting upon the meanings of our perceived wins and fails encourages resilience by recognizing the importance of crucible events in our lives.

How: We are the sum of our physical, mental, and emotional selves, tempered by not only our experiences, but also by how they affect us. By considering the what, why, and how of our events unfolding and resolving, we gain insight. Take the opportunity to review whether they concluded as expected or not, and why. This act of reflection will lead you to new perspectives. As your perspectives change, you will be able to nurture what worked and prune what didn't. You can allow and encourage yourself to grow.

Identifying the level of stress you feel before and then after developing the goal and the steps to meet the goal provides you a measure of your progress. We use the subjective units of distress scale (SUDS) to help us subjectively identify our stress level before, and again after, our efforts. By identifying your initial and final stress levels as somewhere between zero (0) and ten (10), we can make it useful by agreeing that 0 corresponds to no stress and 10 to the highest level of stress you have ever experienced. We are working toward having the SUDS value begin to decrease even as soon as we develop a goal statement and the steps to attain the goal. If the SUDS value increases, it is vital to take some time to reassess the goal statement to assure it is attainable. And don't forget to reassess the steps you plan to use to assure that they have been adequately defined and there are a sufficient number. After all, you want to be able to check off each step to help you mark your progress toward reaching your goal.

Goal Setting Skill—Thriving

Pop quiz!! You have absorbed a lot of information. Now, with a dilemma to solve, it's time to see how well all the knowledge serves you.

Rate the stress level you perceive

Analog SUDS	Digital SUDS	Emoji SUDS
Actually, I'm not stressed	0	
A little stressed	1–3	
Somewhat stressed	4–6	
Quite a bit stressed	7–8	
It's really bad	9	
Run and hide!!	10	

Think about what's stressing you out. What might help?

What was the activating event (A) of that previous circumstance?

Is it similar this time?

What consequences (C) resulted before?

Are you worried the same might happen?

Did your perceived beliefs (B) contribute to those previous outcomes?

Are you concerned they might again?

See anything you might try changing?

Try and identify an objective to help you make these changes.

Now it's time to figure out how to get there.

Write out your thriving goal statement and how you plan to get there, step-by-step.

Hint: You can reuse the systems below as suggested approaches.

Now get started! Don't be shy. Go for it!

Have you made any progress?

Rate the stress level you perceive now

Is it lower?

Yes	No
Congratulations!! You did it!! Now you can do this whenever you need it!	What might have gone wrong? Did you figure out all your steps? Did you actually do them all? Did you give yourself enough time? Was the time set aside to connect? Are you impatient and haven't allowed enough time to see change? Give it another try, from the beginning.

Remember these?

An activating event (A) can be anything, including just contemplating challenging our beliefs. However, more often the (A) will be some external event. Whatever the activating event might be, it will precipitate our recall of the consequences (C), which we saw before. Will these memories help us mobilize our resources, or do they become an obstacle for us being able to perform at our peak?

What was your perceived belief (B) to that previous event? With the benefit of hindsight (20/20 of course), did that belief contribute to the previous consequence? Now be truthful with yourself; did things work out the way you wanted? If not, maybe you had been laboring under some self-defeating thoughts. Maybe using them increased your stress and perhaps sabotaged your efforts.

Here, with the ABCs identified, you can reexamine any of those self-defeating thoughts and/or beliefs and decide if you want to reuse them. Maybe you've come up with a more appropriate, perhaps even more useful, belief.

And there you have it! The act of reflection led you to your new perspective. As your perspective changed, you were able to nurture what worked and prune what didn't. You allowed and encouraged yourself to grow. You've thrived!

In this text, we use the SUDS values from before and then after our efforts. However, it is important to note that SUDS is not the only option for measuring change. You are an individual with your own understanding of what might be a more appropriate measurement for your needs. The only thing that matters is that it can provide meaningful feedback with regard to change, or even transformation, resulting from applying the goal-setting process. Perhaps a scale that measures likelihood of completing the task might be more useful. That scale might range from 0 to 10, where 0 corresponds to zero chance of completion and 10 to fully sure of completion. If you were using a likelihood of completion scale, then you would be working toward an increase in the likelihood you would complete your task from pre-measure to post-measure.

WHY THRIVING?

Resiliency is more than just surviving; it is about growing and learning. It is about thriving in the midst of the stresses that exist in our lives. For better or worse, our most profound life lessons involve loss and/or failure. These become the crucible events in our lives where we learn post-traumatic growth. For example, a study found that 61% of the Vietnam War aviators shot down, imprisoned, and tortured by the North Vietnamese noted psychological benefits from their ordeals.[1] Viktor Frankl, author of *Man's Search for Meaning*, observed countless acts of heroism in the concentration camps during the Holocaust of World War II.[2] Warren Bennis, one of the youngest combat infantry officers in the European theatre during WWII, became an international icon in the field of leadership.[3,4]

Trauma can be the basis for social transformation. For instance, Mothers Against Drunk Drivers (MADD) was founded by a mother who lost her daughter to a repeat offender. Other illustrations of the transformative effects of trauma include such organizations as Physicians for Social Responsibility, Vietnam Veterans Against the War, the International Rescue Committee, Mothers and Grandmothers of the Plaza de Mayo, and the Truth and Reconciliation Commission of South Africa.[5]

Who among us has not experienced suffering and loss? If we live long enough we will all endure stresses and tragedies. We will succeed and fail throughout our lives. While some events may knock us to our knees, resilient people accept that fact, find meaning in it, and then use the lessons learned to find greater purpose and wisdom.

Thriving is about being able to adapt to situations, not about how smart or strong we are. Research has clearly shown that those us who are more flexible in our thinking, display grit (i.e., passion and persistence), and have faith in our abilities (self-efficacy) are better able to cope with life stress in healthier and more productive ways.[6,7,8,9] Resilient people are more likely to view stressors as challenges to conquer rather than problems to be endured.

The reality is that most of us are far more resilient than we know (fig. 6–1).[10,11] In fact, there is evidence suggesting that many survivors of traumatic events, even some with PTSD, can and often do respond to those events with great resilience and personal growth in their lives.[12,13,14] Having worked in the field of trauma for more than 40 years, I have seen such evidence of people's ability to integrate their traumas without becoming defined by them in any negative way. In fact, there is a whole field that looks at a phenomenon called post-traumatic growth (PTG).[15,16] PTG refers to the positive behaviors, attitudes, and skills developed by individuals when they have been confronted with traumatic situations. Such growth does not occur as a result of the trauma itself, but as the result of the adaptive skills, behaviors, and attitudes developed in response to their trauma.[17,18,19] The PTG model reminds us that trauma survivors are not impotent victims—even in the greatest adversity, the potential for growth exists.

Are you a victim or survivor? Consider the following characteristics:

Characteristics of victims	Characteristics of survivors
Victims believe that in order to recover from a traumatic event, they must return to who they were before the event. And, typically, the pretrauma self is idealized.	Survivors recognize that the traumatic experience has permanently changed them and that they must learn to accept those changes and grow from them.
Victims maintain thoughts, feelings, and behaviors that result in continuing post-trauma problems.	Survivors understand that certain thoughts, feelings, and behaviors maintain post-traumatic problems and strive to move away from them.
Victims do not accept personal loss, but put their efforts into thoughts of retaliation and retribution.	Survivors accept that trauma means loss and that they can't turn back the clock. Instead, they work to make new gains and develop an accepting, even forgiving, attitude.
Victims only feel comfortable in the company of other trauma sufferers.	Survivors enjoy their relationships with other survivors, those who understand what others cannot, but they do not do so to the exclusion of other relationships.
Victims can only find negatives in their trauma experiences.	Survivors are able to find opportunities for growth in their traumatic experience. They use those opportunities to build hope and a personal sense of well-being.
Victims use their traumatic experiences as justification for continuing self-destructive thoughts and behaviors. They blame others for their current difficulties.	Survivors understand that they have the power to work to overcome any self-destructive and self-defeating thoughts and behaviors they might have.
Victims have excessive self-blame/guilt relative to their traumatic experiences. They engage in a lot of "should have," "could have," and "if only" kinds of thinking. They are often judgmental and self-condemning.	Survivors accept that they did the best they could in a difficult situation. They are able to have compassion for themselves. Even more important is their ability to use more accurate thinking about themselves relative to their traumatic experience.
Victims discount other people's suffering by comparing traumas. They tend to think that their personal traumas outweigh those of others.	Survivors are able to demonstrate sensitivity to other kinds and others' experiences of personal suffering.

None of us fits completely into one side or the other of this chart and those of us who have been exposed to trauma know that some days are better than others. The point here is that we have a choice to practice the skills required to be more resilient or to surrender and let old ways of thinking and behaving continue to rule our lives. While the events will remain the same, it is in our power to decide the meaning of those events and what we do with them.

Fall seven times, stand up eight.

— Japanese proverb

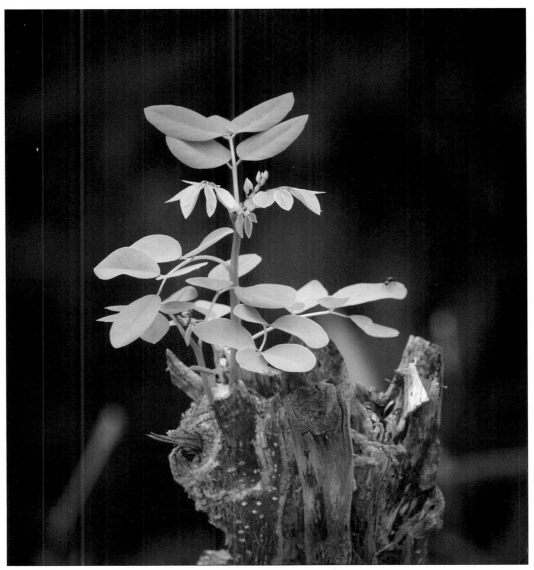

Fig. 6–1. Most of us are far more resilient that we know. (unsplash.com)

THE HOW OF THRIVING

We all grow up and develop *schemas*, which are ways we organize our reality to explain the world, ourselves, and others.[20] Sometimes these schemas become so ingrained that they become stereotypes and lead us into a rigid mind-set.[21,22]

There are number of skills we can use to foster and increase our resilience. Practicing mindfulness, monitoring our thoughts and their impact on our feelings and behavior, and recognizing our strengths are all tools we can use to increase our understanding of ourselves and our ability to have a resilient mind-set.[23,24,25] Sadly, most of us have a hard time focusing on our strengths. We have been taught that to do so is self-centered and self-indulgent. We fall into old traps of self-defeating thoughts about how we, others, and the world should be. But it is our strengths that attract others to us and provide us a healthy understanding of our place in our tribe.[26,27]

Focusing on personal strengths plays a critical role in learning resilience.[28,29,30] Identifying and acknowledging our strengths can help us become more *self-efficacious*,[31] with the belief that we are capable of performing in a certain way to achieve a certain goal. Those with positive self-talk and a belief in themselves are able to persist when faced with challenges.[32,33,34,35] In other words, they are more resilient.

Athletes frequently use positive self-talk to improve their performance.[36,37] We've all watched pregame warm-ups. Do you think they are telling themselves how bad they are going to do and how stupid they are? Probably not!

Self-efficacy is also important in academic performance and can be predictive of whether someone will stay in school.[38,39,40] Resilient people are more likely to graduate from high school, trade school, and/or college, and with higher grades.[41] While the study of self-efficacy is somewhat complex, including in academic settings,[42,43] it is clear that focusing on our strengths can help us become more resilient.[44,45,46]

When we understand that our thoughts and beliefs are what create and how we see ourselves, other people, and the world, we then can construct the kind of world view we want to live in. While this may sound Pollyannaish, recall that resilient people are not unrealistically optimistic or naive. The more we understand our beliefs and thought patterns, the better we will be able to challenge them. It is this that will then help us become more resilient. Some of our core beliefs are positive and adaptive in that they help increase our sense of happiness and satisfaction.[47,48] Other beliefs are maladaptive and harmful to us.[49,50,51] For example, if we have a core belief that says, "If I don't do things perfectly, I'm a failure," then we are doomed, because no one can be perfect. However, the famous Hall of Fame basketball player Michael Jordan suggests another perspective: "I've failed over and over and over again in my life and that is why I succeed."

Jordan's core belief recognizes that failure is a part of life and that success comes from continuing to make the effort, not from berating oneself (or others) for the inability to be perfect. He also said, "I can accept failure, but I can't accept not trying." Again, a core belief for him is that it was the effort that counted, not the outcome. In the world of psychology there is the saying, "Trying is not a behavior." Imagine if Michael Jordan had believed that failure is a sign of weakness and inadequacy. Where would he be?

Do, or do not. There is no "try."

— Yoda

It is in our setbacks that we learn to bounce back. It is in the struggles that confront us that we learn to overcome. It is in the crucible of adversity that we learn to be resilient.

Some people have core beliefs that contend they must always be in control and able to solve their problems on their own. There are many movie characters who teach us that this is the way everyone must be. To be competent we have to be macho; we can't lose control and cry when we are sad or are overwhelmed with joy. Not only must we try to control situations and their outcomes, but we must always be in control of ourselves. If we are unable to be all of those things, we may view ourselves as inadequate. To always be in control also requires us to be ever vigilant, both of others and ourselves. But doing so forces us to deny ourselves the enjoyment of letting others steer the ship, of relaxing and watching life unfold.

Have you ever planned a trip and enjoyed the anticipation of making the journey, imagining all the things that you wanted to see, all the things you were going to do? However, as always happens in life, not everything goes according to how you planned. There are troubles and there are humorous events, even unexpected meetings with others. People who always have to be in control fail to enjoy these surprises. They are unable to go with the flow or enjoy the ride. And later when you look back on the trip, what are the things you remember? Are they of the trip you planned in your mind or the unexpected events, both good and bad? How often in recalling and retelling the story of your trip do you have a good laugh about those occurrences? Yet, at the time, they may have been monumental and caused you frustration and anger because things weren't going as you planned. The situation remained the same, but your thoughts and beliefs have changed. As a consequence, so have your feelings and attitudes.

Another tool for *thriving* is to give new meaning to the traumas and put them into action (fig. 6–2). I've mentioned MADD as an example of the transformative power of taking action after a traumatic event. Other examples from the veteran community include The Mission Continues[52] and Team Rubicon,[53] which recognize the wartime experiences survived as opportunities to continue to be of service to the greater community.

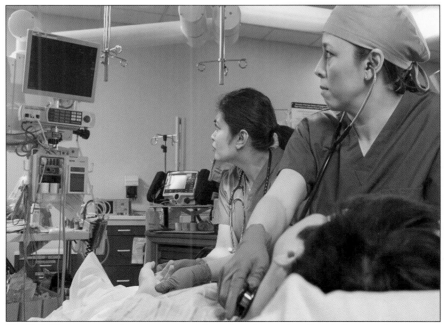

Fig. 6–2. Give new meaning to traumas and put them into action. (istockphoto.com)

Now, let's consider your own beliefs about success and failure, winning and losing, and how they either help you thrive in the midst of stress or how they only lead to obstacles.

▨ Beliefs that help me be more resilient:

_____

_____

_____

_____

▨ Beliefs that get in my way:

_____

_____

_____

_____

▨ What can I do to improve my belief system to increase my resilience?

_____

_____

_____

_____

Defeat is not the worst of failures. Not to have tried is the true failure.

— George Edward Woodberry

INTERNALIZE THRIVING

Recall in as much detail as possible a past personal experience where you practiced something like thriving. That is, a situation where you consciously thought about what belief or attitude was in play when you were dealing with a wins-and-fails type of experience. Given that experience, translate it to the thriving skill. If you prefer, consider writing about your thriving experience as a brief story and build in the thriving skill. Work on this process individually or with others.

Internalizing Worksheet

Remember personal situations you realize led to personal growth and belief in yourself.

Thinking carefully, what did you see as the issue(s) and problem(s) that needed to be addressed?

Identify, as best you can, that dilemma:

What were your fears?

What was evoking those fears?

How likely did you think these would create the feared conclusion(s)?

Did you see this as an adversity?   Why?

Did you see this as an opportunity?   Why?

When you start to review your thoughts:

What was your baseline SUDS?

How did this situation fit with what you had endured before?

Did thinking about this change your SUDS?   Why?

Now, the what, where, and how:

Think about how you were holding yourself hostage.

What does this reveal about your beliefs at the time?

Should you have reconsidered those beliefs?

What alternative conclusion(s) did you want?

How did you encourage it?

Think about how likely this option seemed.

How long did you commit?

After you review these steps, what was your resulting SUDS:

Do you think you might have used any of our other skills?

Which ones?

Now let's think about whether all this will help:

Did this process make your impression of the event more manageable?   How?

Did this process make your impression of the event more compelling?   How?

Can you think of anything to change in this skill to make it more personally useful?

How about the future? Do you think you will be able to put your results to the test?

Do you think you will be able to reliably enable successful results?   Why?

In training events when I ask others to recall an event where they feel that they thrived, I am reminded of a multitude of situations in my life where I have used this important skill. What I remember most vividly was a high school counselor telling me that I wasn't smart enough to attend college. I could have easily accepted his assessment, but chose to use it as motivation to get my Ph.D.

He conquers who endures.

— Persius

EXTERNALIZE: APPLY THRIVING AS A GROUP

Case Study: You are completing some paperwork after responding to a vehicular accident involving a child. You notice your partner is visibly agitated. You are aware that your partner responded to an incident last week where a disoriented child had wandered onto the highway and had been hit multiple times. Your partner admits to having some difficulty dealing with this current incident and asks if you have any suggestions.

How might you respond to this situation? Your goal is to use thriving to develop a potential solution. And don't be shy about using any of the others skills you think might help.

It is only in your thriving that you have anything to offer anyone.

— Esther Hicks

PRACTICE THRIVING

Practice Worksheet

Remember personal situations you realize led to personal growth and belief in yourself.

Identify, as best you can, the current dilemma:

> What are your fears?
>
> What is evoking those fears?
>
> How likely do you think these will create the feared conclusion(s)?
>
> Do you see this as an adversity? Why?
>
> Do you see this as an opportunity? Why?

When you start to review your thoughts:

> What is your baseline SUDS?
>
> How does this situation fit with what you had endured before?
>
> Does thinking about this change your SUDS? Why?

Now, the what, where, and how:

> Think about how you are holding yourself hostage.
>
> > Does it seem familiar?
>
> What does this reveal about your perspective or your beliefs at this time?
>
> > Should you reconsider those?
>
> What alternative conclusion(s) do you want?
>
> > How did you encourage it before?
>
> > How will you encourage it now?
>
> Think about how likely this option seems.
>
> How long will you commit?

After you review these steps, what is your resulting SUDS:

Do you think you might use any of our other skills?

Which ones?

Now let's think about whether all this will help:

Does this process make your impression of the event more manageable?   How?

Does this process make your impression of the event more compelling?   How?

Can you think of anything to change in this skill to make it more personally useful?

This is your future. Now it's time to put your results to the test:

Do you think you will be able to reliably enable successful results?   Why?

Resilience is all about being able to overcome the unexpected.
Sustainability is about survival.
The goal of resilience is to thrive.

— Jamais Cascio

APPLY THRIVING TO A COMMUNITY

Define the community (family, social support group, team, organization, or neighborhood) where you are intending to apply the skill, why this skill is appropriate for the particular community, and how the skill would be administered. What techniques might you use to introduce the concept of thriving and what would be your specific expectation of the outcome? Are you aware of a community situation that you can apply to the thriving mind-set?

> *Salvatore Maddi tells the story about a situation they had investigated in their early research on hardiness in which an entire HR department had been let go by Illinois Bell. Rather than being immobilized by this devastating news, the HR director and some of the former employees established their own human resources company. According to the story, a few years later Illinois Bell approached this highly successful HR company to contract with them to fulfill their HR needs. They had thrived so well, they couldn't take the offer and had to refer them to other resources.*[54]

You're braver than you believe,
and stronger than you seem,
and smarter than you think.

— A.A. Milne

REMEMBERING THRIVING

Again, take the opportunity now to reflect on the skill and associate some key words or phrases that help to succinctly define the skill of thriving, using your own words (fig. 6–3). When you have completed this process, compare these key words and phrases with the person or persons with whom you are working. Discuss and decide if you wish to alter any of your reflective key words or phrases. What have you learned through this process?

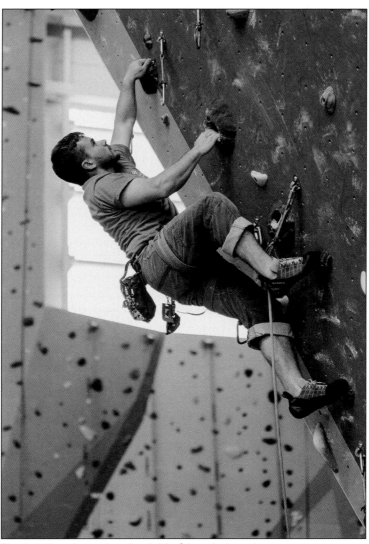

Fig. 6–3. How do you describe thriving? (unsplash.com)

NOTES

1. Tedeschi, Richard G. and Richard J. McNally. "Can we facilitate posttraumatic growth in combat veterans?" *American Psychologist* 66, no. 1 (2011): 19-24.

2. Frankl, Viktor E. *Man's Search for Meaning.* New York: Simon and Schuster, 1985.

3. Bennis, Warren G. *On Becoming a Leader.* New York: Basic Books, 2003.

4. Putman, Paul G. "Strategic Leadership Competency Development." In Wang, Victor C. X. *Encyclopedia of Strategic Leadership and Management.* Hershey, PA: IGI Global, 2017, 1495-1520.

5. Bloom, Sandra L. "By the crowd they have been broken, by the crowd they shall be healed: The social transformation of trauma." In Tedeschi, Richard G., Crystal L. Park, and Lawrence G. Calhoun, eds. *Posttraumatic Growth: Positive Changes in the Aftermath of Crisis.* Mahwah, NJ: Lawrence Erlbaum Assoc., 1998, 179-213.

6. Dweck, Carol S. *Mindset: The New Psychology of Success.* New York: Random House Digital, Inc., 2008.

7. Duckworth, Angela. *Grit: The Power of Passion and Perseverance.* New York: Simon and Schuster, 2016.

8. Schwarzer, Ralf, ed. *Self-Efficacy: Thought Control of Action.* Oxfordshire: Taylor & Francis, 2014.

9. Karademas, Evangelos C. "Self-efficacy, social support and well-being: The mediating role of optimism." *Personality and Individual Differences* 40, no. 6 (2006): 1281-1290.

10. Bonanno, George A. "Loss, trauma, and human resilience: Have we underestimated the human capacity to thrive after extremely aversive events?" *American Psychologist* 59, no. 1 (2004): 20-28.

11. Liu, Jenny J. W., Maureen Reed, and Todd A. Girard. "Advancing resilience: An integrative, multi-system model of resilience." *Personality and Individual Differences* 111, no. 1 (2017): 111-118.

12. Bonanno, George A. and Erica D. Diminich. "Annual research review: Positive adjustment to adversity—trajectories of minimal-impact resilience and emergent resilience." *Journal of Child Psychology and Psychiatry* 54, no. 4 (2013): 378-401.

13. Bonanno, George A., Chris R. Brewin, Krzysztof Kaniasty, and Annette M. La Greca. "Weighing the costs of disaster: Consequences, risks, and resilience in individuals, families, and communities." *Psychological Science in the Public Interest* 11, no. 1 (2010): 1-49.

14. Quiros, Laura. "Book review: Trauma, recovery, and growth: Positive psychological perspectives on posttraumatic stress." *Journal of Teaching in Social Work* 30, no. 1 (2010): 118-121.

15. Calhoun, Lawrence G. and Richard G. Tedeschi, eds. *Handbook of Posttraumatic Growth: Research and Practice.* New York: Routledge, 2014.

16. Knobler, Haim Y., H. Knobler, E. Cohen, and M. Z. Abramowitz. "Lessons to be learned from the resilience and post traumatic growth of Holocaust survivors." *European Journal of Public Health* 26, suppl. 1 (2016): ckw171-042.

17. Peterson, Christopher, Nansook Park, Nnamdi Pole, Wendy D'Andrea, and Martin E. P. Seligman. "Strengths of character and posttraumatic growth." *Journal of Traumatic Stress* 21, no. 2 (2008): 214-217.

18. Park, Crystal L., Jennifer Chmielewski, and Thomas O. Blank. "Post-traumatic growth: Finding positive meaning in cancer survivorship moderates the impact of intrusive thoughts on adjustment in younger adults." *Psycho-Oncology* 19, no. 11 (2010): 1139-1147.

19. Karagiorgou, Olga, Jonathan J. Evans, and Breda Cullen. "Post-traumatic growth in adult survivors of brain injury: A qualitative study of participants completing a pilot trial of brief positive psychotherapy." *Disability and Rehabilitation* 40, no. 6 (2017): 1-8.

20. Janoff-Bulman, Ronnie. "Assumptive worlds and the stress of traumatic events: Applications of the schema construct." *Social Cognition* 7, no. 2 (1989): 113-136.

21. Kray, Laura J. and Aiwa Shirako. "Stereotype threat in organizations: An examination of its scope, triggers, and possible interventions." In Inzlicht, Michael and Toni Schmader, eds. *Stereotype Threat: Theory, Process, and Application.* New York: Oxford University Press, 2012, 173-187.

22. Hacker, Stephen. "Courage in the face of nonsense: Leading in the workplace." *Journal for Quality and Participation* 39, no. 4 (2017): 15.

23. Jha, Amishi P., Alexandra B. Morrison, Suzanne C. Parker, and Elizabeth A. Stanley. "Practice is protective: Mindfulness training promotes cognitive resilience in high-stress cohorts." *Mindfulness* 8, no. 1 (2017): 46-58.

24. Goldhagen, Brian E., Karen Kingsolver, Sandra S. Stinnett, and Jullia A. Rosdahl. "Stress and burnout in residents: Impact of mindfulness-based resilience training." *Advances in Medical Education and Practice* 6 (2015): 535-532.

25. Benight, Charles C. and Albert Bandura. "Social cognitive theory of posttraumatic recovery: The role of perceived self-efficacy." *Behaviour Research and Therapy* 42, no. 10 (2004): 1129-1148.

26   Martínez-Martí, María Luisa, and Willibald Ruch. "Character strengths predict resilience over and above positive affect, self-efficacy, optimism, social support, self-esteem, and life satisfaction." *The Journal of Positive Psychology* 12, no. 2 (2017): 110-119.

27   Snyder, Charles R., Shane J. Lopez, and Jennifer Teramoto Pedrotti. *Positive Psychology: The Scientific and Practical Explorations of Human Strengths*. Los Angeles: Sage Publications, 2010.

28   Escandón, Socorro, Martha L. Martinez, and Jacquelyn H. Flaskerud. "Exploring character strengths: Forging a relationship between nursing students and community youth." *Issues in Mental Health Nursing* 37, no. 11 (2016): 875-877.

29   Tedeschi, Richard G. and Ryan P. Kilmer. "Assessing strengths, resilience, and growth to guide clinical interventions." *Professional Psychology: Research and Practice* 36, no. 3 (2005): 230-237.

30   Seibert, Scott E., Maria L. Kraimer, and Peter A. Heslin. "Developing career resilience and adaptability." *Organizational Dynamics* 3, no. 45 (2016): 245-257.

31   Rashid, Tayyab, Ruth Louden, Laurie Wright, Ron Chu, Aryel Maharaj, Irfan Hakim, Danielle Uy, and Bruce Kidd. "Flourish: A strengths-based approach to building student resilience." In Proctor, Carmel, ed. *Positive Psychology Interventions in Practice*. Cham: Springer International Publishing, 2017, 29-45.

32   Bandura, Albert. "Self-efficacy: Toward a unifying theory of behavioral change." *Psychological Review* 84, no. 2 (1977): 191-125.

33   Warner, Lisa M., Benjamin Schüz, Julia K. Wolff, Linda Parschau, Susanne Wurm, and Ralf Schwarzer. "Sources of self-efficacy for physical activity." *Health Psychology* 33, no. 11 (2014): 1298-1308.

34   Hardy, James. "Speaking clearly: A critical review of the self-talk literature." *Psychology of Sport and Exercise* 7, no. 1 (2006): 81-97.

35   Barratt, Caroline. "Exploring how mindfulness and self-compassion can enhance compassionate care." *Nursing Standard* 31, no. 21 (2017): 55-63.

36   Hardy, James, Craig R. Hall, and Mike R. Alexander. "Exploring self-talk and affective states in sport." *Journal of Sports Sciences* 19, no. 7 (2001): 469-475.

37   Rogerson, Lisa J. and Dennis W. Hrycaiko. "Enhancing competitive performance of ice hockey goaltenders using centering and self-talk." *Journal of Applied Sport Psychology* 14, no. 1 (2002): 14-26.

38   Bong, Mimi. "Role of self-efficacy and task-value in predicting college students' course performance and future enrollment intentions." *Contemporary Educational Psychology* 26, no. 4 (2001): 553-570.

39   Hidi, Suzanne and Judith M. Harackiewicz. "Motivating the academically unmotivated: A critical issue for the 21st century." *Review of Educational Research* 70, no. 2 (2000): 151-179.

40   Taylor, Heidi and Helen Reyes. "Self-efficacy and resilience in baccalaureate nursing students." *International Journal of Nursing Education Scholarship* 9, no. 1 (2012): 1-13.

41   Lifton, Donald E., Sandara Seay, and Andrew Bushko. "Can student 'hardiness' serve as an indicator of likely persistence to graduation? Baseline results from a longitudinal study." *Academic Exchange Quarterly* 4, no. 2 (2000): 73-81.

42   Pintrich, Paul R. "A conceptual framework for assessing motivation and self-regulated learning in college students." *Educational Psychology Review* 16, no. 4 (2004): 385-407.

43   Wolters, Christopher A., Shirley L. Yu, and Paul R. Pintrich. "The relation between goal orientation and students' motivational beliefs and self-regulated learning." *Learning and Individual Differences* 8, no. 3 (1996): 211-238.

44   Butler, Courtney, Courtney Watford, Shamanda S. Burston, James P. Morgan, and David Carscaddon. "Positive counseling with college students." *Journal of Counseling and Psychology* 1, no. 1 (2016): 1.

45   Hass, Michael, Quaylan Allen, and Michelle Amoah. "Turning points and resilience of academically successful foster youth." *Children and Youth Services Review* 44 (2014): 387-392.

46   Robertson, Ivan T., Cary L. Cooper, Mustafa Sarkar, and Thomas Curran. "Resilience training in the workplace from 2003 to 2014: A systematic review." *Journal of Occupational and Organizational Psychology* 88, no. 3 (2015): 533-562.

47   Whiteside, Mary, Komla Tsey, Yvonne Cadet-James, and Janya McCalman. "Beliefs and attitudes." In *Promoting Aboriginal Health: The Family Wellbeing Empowerment Approach*. Cham: Springer International Publishing, 2014, 19-24.

48   Joshanloo, Mohsen, Yeong Ock Park, and Sang Hee Park. "Optimism as the moderator of the relationship between fragility of happiness beliefs and experienced happiness." *Personality and Individual Differences* 106 (2017): 61-63.

49   Wong, Quincy J. J., Peter M. McEvoy, and Ronald M. Rapee. "A comparison of repetitive negative thinking and post-event processing in the prediction of maladaptive social-evaluative beliefs: A short-term prospective study." *Journal of Psychopathology and Behavioral Assessment* 38, no. 2 (2016): 230-241.

50   Caselli, Gabriele, Alessia Offredi, Francesca Martino, Davide Varalli, Giovanni M. Ruggiero, Sandra Sassaroli, Marcantonio M. Spada, and Adrian Wells. "Metacognitive beliefs and rumination as predictors of anger: A prospective study." *Aggressive Behavior* 43, no. 5 (2017): 421-429.

51   Kloss, Jacqueline D., Christina O. Nash, Colleen M. Walsh, Elizabeth Culnan, Sarah Horsey, and Kathy Sexton-Radek. "A 'Sleep 101' program for college students improves sleep hygiene knowledge and reduces maladaptive beliefs about sleep." *Behavioral Medicine* 42, no. 1 (2016): 48-56.

52   The Mission Continues. https://www.missioncontinues.org.

53   Team Rubicon. https://teamrubiconusa.org.

54   Maddi, Salvatore R. *Hardiness Training*. Irvine: University of California, Irvine, 2006.

7

EMPATHY

Could a greater miracle take place than for us
to look through each other's eyes for an instant?

— Henry David Thoreau

OVERVIEW

Why: Empathy is the capacity to understand what another being is experiencing from within the other being's frame of reference. Empathy allows one to understand and anticipate the actions of others. Empathy provides opportunity to reach out and foster communication.

How: To "put yourself in another's shoes" is an often-quoted foundational consideration to experience empathy. To encourage it, do the following:

- Recognize your own biases and emotions.
- Interact with a wide range of people with different backgrounds.
- Be curious about the similarities and differences between yourself and others.
- Ask others for their point of view.
- Listen without offering advice.
- Read good fiction.
- Cultivate your imagination.

Identifying a measure of change between before and then after developing the goal and the steps to meet the goal provides us with a way to measure our success. Here, we suggest the use of SUDS to help you subjectively identify your stress levels before setting a goal, and again after the goal is attained. The levels are somewhere between zero (0) and ten (10), where 0 corresponds to no stress and 10 to the highest level of stress you have ever experienced. The anticipation is that the SUDS level begins to decrease even after developing a goal statement and the steps to attain the goal. If your SUDS level increases, then take some time to reassess your goal statement to assure it is attainable. And reassess the steps to assure that they have been adequately defined and there are as many as you need. After all, you want to be able to check off each step and mark progress toward reaching your goal.

Goal Setting Skill—Empathy

Just as stress affects you, so too does stress affect others. As you think about this, do you care?

Rate the stress level you perceive

Analog SUDS	Digital SUDS	Emoji SUDS
Actually, I'm not stressed	0	
A little stressed	1–3	
Somewhat stressed	4–6	
Quite a bit stressed	7–8	
It's really bad	9	
Run and hide!!	10	

Think about what's stressing you out. What might help?

Try and identify an objective to help you do that.

Write out an empathy goal statement about how you might look at your dilemmas differently, step-by-step.

Now get started! Don't be shy. Go for it!

Have you made any progress?

Rate the stress level you perceive now

Is it lower?

Yes	No
Congratulations!! You did it!! Now you can do this whenever you need it!	What might have gone wrong? Did you figure out all your steps? Did you actually do them all? Did you give yourself enough time? Was the time set aside to connect? Are you impatient and haven't allowed enough time to see change?

Is SUDS the only option for measuring change? Certainly not! You are encouraged to find the most appropriate measurement for your needs. The only thing that matters is that it can provide meaningful feedback with regard to change, or even transformation, resulting from applying the goal-setting process. Perhaps a scale that measures the likelihood of completing the task might be more useful. That scale might range from 0 to 10, where 0 corresponds to zero chance of completion and 10 is fully sure of completion. If you were using a likelihood-of-completion scale, then you would anticipate an increase in likelihood to complete from premeasure to postmeasure.

We are all veterans of something.

— Greg Burham, Navy SEAL, Vietnam

WHY EMPATHY?

We often confuse empathy and sympathy[1,2] but they are quite different.[3] *Empathy* denotes understanding. *Sympathy* also indicates understanding, but it goes further. Sympathy incorporates agreement, support, even approval. Empathy does not.

Empathy is a survival skill. Ask any combat veteran about getting ready to go outside the wire and they will tell you at some point they began thinking about what the enemy was doing and planning. They were empathizing with the enemy. Ask any police officer or first responder about coming upon a scene and they will tell you that in order to maintain control over the scene they need to empathize with the people involved.

Empathy is the capacity to understand what someone else is experiencing from within the other's frame of reference. It allows us to understand and anticipate both the other person's and our own actions. Empathy provides us an opportunity to reach out and foster communication. Empathy also helps us become better critical thinkers,[4,5,6] which is imperative to support our decision making and a critical skill for those of us who are care providers.[7,8,9]

Now, what do you think is necessary to metamorphose into a critical-thinking butterfly? Research shows that we need to develop the following intellectual characteristics to become critical thinkers:[10]

- Intellectual humility
- Intellectual courage
- Intellectual empathy
- Intellectual integrity
- Intellectual perseverance
- Faith in reason
- A strong sense of justice

To be a critical thinker requires us to have the courage to be open to another viewpoint. We must be able to suspend judgment, to avoid black-and-white thinking. The clarity, the meaning that we give to situations and words, both in ourselves and others, is crucial. Thus, the goal of critical thinking, and a success trait for any professional, is to distinguish fact from opinion, determine the reliability of the source, and distinguish the accuracy and relevancy of that information. Identifying bias and unstated assumptions and recognizing logical inconsistencies are the characteristics that will help us succeed.

Research has demonstrated that empathy can increase positive clinical outcomes.[11,12,13] Sadly, it has been reported that there is a decline in empathy among medical students.[14,15] However, efforts like this text and other works are attempting to help care providers understand the benefits of empathy for themselves, their families, and their patients.[16,17,18]

Resilient people understand that they can't do it alone. Recognizing and developing the ability to reach out encourages the establishing of a social support system. Reaching out and seeking help is a complex process. How do we recognize when do we need to reach out, and where? We are faced with anticipating the attitudes and beliefs of any person who may be offering us help. That and more has to be considered under the cloud of the issue under consideration.[19,20] Unfortunately, care providers are not the best at reaching out. Many (often unconsciously) are poor in engaging in other available and appropriate self-care behaviors.[21,22,23]

Compounding this is the fact that there are significant differences between men and women in their attitudes and behaviors about reaching out to others.[24,25,26,27] To make matters worse, health care cultures can discourage reaching out by regarding such behavior as weak or a sign of incompetence.[28,29,30] Simply put, we need to take care of ourselves before we can take care of others. Put another way, everyone, and especially caregivers, needs to model the behaviors we want others, including our family members, our colleagues, and our communities, to integrate into their lives.[31,32]

Interestingly, there is recent research that demonstrates the power of vulnerability.[33,34] In fact, some studies have shown that when we practice and refine the ability to reach out and be vulnerable to others we develop reasonable trust instead of enduring blind trust and gullibility (fig. 7–1).[35,36] Rather than always being a negative trait, being vulnerable can improve our relationships. Being vulnerable helps build our trust in ourselves and others, and it improves our ability to empathize.[37]

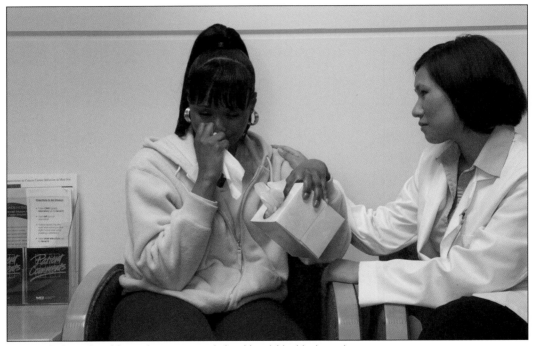

Fig. 7–1. Being vulnerable can improve our relationships. (videoblock.com)

Empathy is an important characteristic of resilient people.[38,39,40] Empathy is the ability to recognize what someone else is going through. Empathy does not require agreement with the other person's point of view but instead entails understanding it. As mentioned earlier, this is a crucial survival skill. It supports our ability to interpret another's state of mind. Such an association, in its role in helping anticipate another's future responses and actions, plays a crucial part of preparing yourself for any situation.

Many of us have been taught that empathy is a weakness and we have to be strong in the midst of suffering.[41] Yet, resilient people are curious about things, including how to gain understanding of another's point of view. By understanding every perspective, they choose to become more empathic. They are also willing to challenge themselves to explore obstacles both inside and outside themselves that impede their abilities.

Empathy requires us to have a flexible mindset. Further, it has been shown to increase organizational effectiveness by encouraging collaboration.[42,43,44] Even in the development of the critical thinking, empathy has been found to be essential.[45,46,47]

THE HOW OF EMPATHY

One of the first things we need to understand is that each and every one of us has our own personal thoughts and biases about being empathic. These beliefs about empathy can either enhance or hinder our ability to become more resilient. The ability to see from a different perspective is considered a cornerstone of resilience by some authors.[48,49,50]

Reflect: What thoughts, feelings, and beliefs do you have when you think about the terms "empathy" or "reaching out"? Do these beliefs increase or decrease your stress level?

Anything else? Of course! Along with understanding your own thoughts and emotions, consider the following skills to increase your empathy:

Empathy Skills

- Interact with a wide range of people with different backgrounds.
- Look at the similarities between yourself and others.
- Practice taking on another's point of view.
- Listen to others without offering advice and really hear them.
- Be open to receiving empathy from others.
- Forgive others.
- Read good fiction.
- Laugh at yourself.

Case Study: Your friend's wife is frustrated, if not a bit annoyed. His commitment to his schooling and his part-time job is leaving her feeling too far removed. He decides he will purposefully focus on improving his empathy. As a group discussion and to familiarize ourselves with the empathy worksheet, which skills should he include and how might we develop this skill to help him?

What is the current situation?

▨ What empathy skill(s) might be useful?

_____
_____

▨ Why?

_____
_____
_____
_____

Here is another exercise that you can do to understand the importance of empathy, critical thinking, and seeing from another person's point of view:

- Try standing back-to-back with another individual. Looking straight ahead, describe what you see. Have the other individual describe what he or she sees.

▨ Who is correct? Why?

_____
_____
_____
_____

▨ What can you learn from this exercise?

_____
_____
_____
_____

COMMUNICATION

We have two ears and one mouth so that we can listen
twice as much as we speak.

—Epictetus

We are herd animals and our mutual survival is dependent on others, just as they are dependent on us. With rare exceptions, we cannot survive alone and our development is dependent on social interaction.[51,52,53] We need to belong to a tribe, a group, a family, a squad, or a community.[54] It may be tempting to say that we would like to be left alone, but for most of us we would soon long for human contact. Learning to live successfully in a group can be challenging and requires a great deal of patience and commitment. Learning how to communicate effectively is vital to effective personal interactions and to becoming resilient. One of the more important aspects of communicating effectively is the ability to empathize with the people you are communicating with. Again, to empathize does not necessarily mean you agree with the other person's point of view. Rather, just as with the exercise above, the effort is to understand the other's point of view.

It is also crucial to recognize some of the important elements of communication. It has been proposed that most of human communication is nonverbal, perhaps as much as two-thirds.[55,56] While there are some cultural differences, our communication includes body language, voice tone, facial expressions, and eye contact.

The following is an example I witnessed when I was the director of a PTSD outpatient clinic at the Southern Arizona VA Health Care System.

Case study: Two colleagues were discussing an earlier encounter with another person and both had a different viewpoint of what was going on with that person. Early in the discussion, both colleagues were amiable and collegial. Each was listening to the other. A bit later, one of the individuals crossed his arms and began to puff up his chest as he was making a point. Almost immediately, the other individual began to talk louder and more argumentatively and the conversation ended with both of them abruptly walking away. When asked later, both recalled the puffing-up as the point where the discussion turned into an argument. It was not the words but the behavior that changed the tone.

To become effective communicators, we need to learn to be aware of nonverbal behaviors, no matter from whom. We can, for example, communicate the wrong message by our body language. We can also be reacting to nonverbal cues and not actually hearing the words of others. If we can monitor our reactions to other people's nonverbal behaviors, then we can improve the accuracy of our thinking, a trait of a resilient person.

Reflect: What are your thoughts about listening to others and about being listened to?

_____

_____

_____

_____

Men, for the most part, communicate to impart information and to solve problems. Women generally communicate to connect with other people.[57] Not understanding this difference, and its empathic implications, can lead to a lot of stress and conflict in relationships. A husband may complain that his wife is nagging him with questions, but her efforts are really an attempt to connect with him. Perhaps a wife comes to her husband with a problem that she wants to share with him. She is probably more than capable of solving the problem herself, but the husband hears this as a problem for him to solve. As a consequence, he interrupts his wife, offers his solution, and goes on about his business feeling good about how smart he is at fixing the problem. He is then baffled by his wife's cold silence. Why would she react this way when he had come up with such a brilliant solution? Because it was her need to connect with him, not have him solve her problem.

Men, unfortunately, are not always the best listeners and in conversation will interrupt far more often than women.[58] These differences between male and female communication have been humorously acknowledged as men compartmentalizing topics and women seeing connections.[59] A great example of this behavior is illustrated in the video *It's Not about the Nail*.[60] For me, it hit the nail on the head; it truly drove the point home. Okay, bad puns, but to understand why these are so bad, you'll have to watch it!

Reflect: *Silent* is an anagram of *listen*; both words use the same letters. Is this a coincidence? Many of us have been in situations where we were listening to someone and, after the first two sentences, we began to compose our response without listening to the remainder of the other's contribution. We have also been on the receiving end of this same treatment.

Reflect: When you become aware another individual has disconnected, what is your first thought? What were the cues you observed?

_____

_____

_____

_____

Sadly, there is data that shows that health care providers are not the best listeners.[61,62] Thankfully, though, listening is a skill that can be learned.[63] Effective listeners make the best communicators because they are aware of what their audience wants and needs from them; they hear the words as well as the message associated with the words (fig. 7–2).

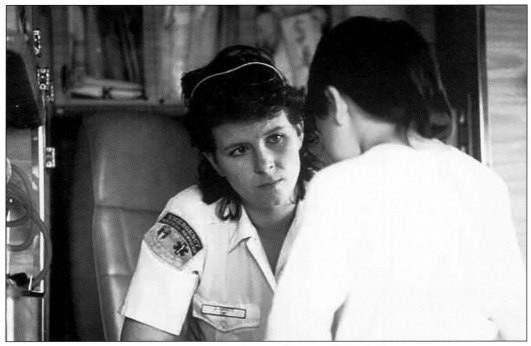

Fig. 7–2. Effective listeners make the best communicators. (Courtesy of Mike Grill.)

Here is an exercise that is frequently used in marriage counseling to help couples improve their listening skills, called ticket-to-talk. Take one 3×5 card, or perhaps a coffee cup or some small article. The person with the card—the ticket—is the only one who can talk. When that individual is finished talking, the other must paraphrase back to the individual with the ticket what they heard. The individual with the ticket determines the accuracy of the response. If it is accurate, then the ticket switches to the other person. If not, then the individual with the ticket restates their message. The listener then makes another attempt at paraphrasing. (Obviously, when you have the ticket, keep your message succinct to keep the process manageable.)

Reflect: If you are in a resilience training course and you are using the TAPPS approach, also known as a collaborative group approach, practice ticket-to-talk. After the exercise, discuss what this reveals about how you might go about improving your listening skills. If you are working on this skill and want to practice it later, think about who you want to run through this exercise with. Either way, share with the group what you observed and learned about yourself.

FIGHTING

We all would like to live in relationships where there is no conflict. This is, however, unrealistic optimism and such a fantasy does not teach us to be resilient. Fighting, whether in disagreements, arguments, or conflicts, is a part of the human condition. We all have diverse backgrounds, life experiences, and perspectives. Rather than seeing this as a negative, we can elect to see it as an opportunity to learn about ourselves and other people.

Everyone has individual beliefs about fighting, and these beliefs impact how we fight. Some people feel that they have to win an argument at any cost, even if it means the end of a relationship. Other people will be more passive-aggressive in their fighting style and appear to acquiesce, only to ambush the person at another time or about another topic. One method of looking at these interactions is through what can be termed *communication filters*, which are factors that affect the sender and receiver. Five communication filters have been identified that can impact our ability to communicate effectively in times of conflict:[64]

Communication Filters

- External and internal distractions
- Emotional states
- Beliefs and expectations
- Differences in communication styles
- Self-protection or fear of being rejected

Each of these filters has an impact on our effectiveness and resilience in the midst of conflict. For example, if our belief is that we must defend or protect ourselves when someone says something hurtful to us or makes us afraid, then we may be limiting ourselves to an emotional state such as anger.

Our thoughts and beliefs can profoundly impact how we perceive a situation. For example, someone who is already hypervigilant, continually tense, and on guard may be even more vulnerable to overreacting to inconsequential remarks.

If we believe that conflict is to be avoided at all costs because we are afraid of our reaction or being rejected, then we will build up resentment toward others where there is conflict.

We can often prevent conflict from escalating by becoming good empathic listeners. It has been suggested that in conflict or difficult conversations, there are three different elements going on at the same time: what happened, feelings, and identity.[65]

- The first element is the *what happened* or *what should have happened* conversation, where the conflict usually has to do with whose viewpoint is "right" and whose viewpoint is "wrong." There are generally lots of should and would statements, as well as finger pointing.

- The second element is the *feelings* conversation, with emerging questions such as "Am I justified in feeling this way?" or "Are the other person's feelings valid?" It is important to recognize the feelings conversation because if ignored, the feelings will surface at some later time. Have you ever been ambushed by someone who didn't express or admit what they were feeling in a previous conflict, only to bring it up again at a later time?

- The third element is the *identity* conversation, which can be described as an internal debate over whether this means we are competent or incompetent, a good or bad person, worthy of love or unlovable. This interaction includes questions about our self-worth and self-image.

No one deals completely, effectively, and simultaneously with these three different elements of conversations. Rather, a realistic goal is to have a working knowledge of what happens in a conflict so you are not as likely to be blindsided or overreact, because this could easily escalate the situation.

Most of us just want to be listened to and understood. If we can communicate effectively and empathetically, we have gone a long way to de-escalating a potential conflict. Conversely, if we become caustic, demeaning, and belittling of someone's thoughts and perceptions, then we only fuel the fight. When you are in conflict with someone else, consider these questions:[66]

- Would I want anyone to talk to me the way I am speaking to others?

- How would others describe me as I communicate with them?

- What makes it easier for me to listen to others?

- What do others say or do that turns me off and keeps me from listening to their message?

Another way to interpret communications is through interactions.[67,68] Consider the following four ways that humans communicate with each other:

- *Aggressively*, where the aggressor's feelings count and the passive person's do not.

- *Passively*, where the other person's feelings count and those of the passive person don't.

- *Assertively*, where my feelings count and so do yours.

- *Passive-aggressively*, where one person pretends to acknowledge the other person's feelings.

The most effective way of communicating with someone, especially when we are fighting, is to do so assertively.[69]

Reflect: Is it more important for you to be right, or to resolve the differences between you and another person? Why?

_____

_____

_____

_____

You might also consider watching the older movie version of *Twelve Angry Men*, especially the chapter of the eyewitness (approximately 6 minutes). If you are working with a group, use the TAPPS collaborative group discussions to interpret the personal communication from the movie. Pay particular attention to the four ways humans communicate. Based on a character in the movie or upon yourself, attempt to respond to the following questions.

Checklist for Internalizing Empathy

Can you think of a situation where you benefited from the empathy skill?

Thinking carefully, what do you see as the issue(s) and need(s) that must be addressed?

Identify, as best you can, the dilemma you face:

   Do you remember having any fears about working with other people?

   Do you remember having any thoughts about the possible gains from such cooperation?

   What does this reveal about your beliefs at the time?

   Did you reconsider those beliefs?

   Did you see this as an adversity?   Why?

   Did you see this as an opportunity?   Why?

When you started to review your plans, what was your baseline SUDS:

SUDS intensity (0–10)

   How did this situation fit with what you had thought about before?   Why?

   Did thinking about this change your SUDS?   Why?

Now, the what, where, and how:

   Think about how you were holding yourself hostage.

   What alternative conclusion(s) did you want?

   How did you encourage it?

   Think about how likely this option seemed.

   How did your formalizing your approach help?

After you review these perspectives, what is your resulting SUDS:

   SUDS intensity (0–10)

Do you think you might have used any of our other skills?

Which ones?

Now let's think about whether all this helped:

Did writing the goal statement make the task clearer?

Did writing the goal statement make the task more manageable?

Did writing the steps needed make the task clearer?

Did writing the steps needed make the task more manageable?

Was checking off each step as it was completed helpful?

Did this process make your impression of the event more compelling?

Can you think of anything you might change in this skill to make it more personally useful?

How about the future? Do you think you will be able to put your results to the test?

Reflect: What methods did you personally use that demonstrated empathy?

_____

_____

_____

_____

What methods did someone else use that demonstrated empathy?

_____

_____

_____

_____

What were the consequences that made this event memorable?

_____

_____

_____

_____

What did you learn from this exercise?

_____

_____

_____

_____

EXTERNALIZE: APPLY EMPATHY AS A GROUP

Effective communication takes into account empathy and listening skills. The ability to empathize with the individual or people with whom we are communicating does not require agreement with that other person's point of view. Rather, empathy entails understanding another person's viewpoint. Acknowledging the importance of empathy as foundational to critical thinking, listening, and even fighting fairly is resilience in action. Given these tools, examine the following case study.

Case study: A former work associate who is also an old friend calls you. Though you live fairly close, you have differing work shifts so socializing is very difficult. It has been a few months since you last met. You recall that he was very unhappy with his new employer. He apologizes for not responding to your emails. He mentions that the back pain he had been experiencing was finally diagnosed as a debilitating birth defect. He states that he has been angry and depressed, feeling completely trapped by his life situations. However, you notice that he seems quite upbeat. Surprised, you ask him, "What's up?"

He replies, "Yes. I have decided to make some changes. And that's the reason I am calling you. Would you mind taking care of my dog for a few days? I will leave the key under the mat."

With no hesitation, you tell him, "Of course I will."

When you ask if he is traveling, he tells you, "I'm heading to the mountains to have some alone time. I haven't been sleeping well and I just want to have some quiet and a good long sleep. Oh, and do you remember that prized autographed baseball? Well, it's waiting for you at the house. I really appreciate you taking care of Twinkies."

This is an example of how empathy helps you respond to this situation. How do you feel about your use of empathy to let you clearly understand the situation? Can you think of any other resilience skills that would also be helpful?

_____

_____

_____

_____

Checklist for Externalizing Empathy

Can you think of a situation where you might benefit from the empathy skill?

Thinking carefully, what did you see as the issue(s) and need(s) that had to be addressed?

Identify, as best you can, the dilemma you face:

Do you have any fears about working with other people?

Do you have any thoughts about the possible gains from such cooperation?

What does this reveal about your beliefs?

Should you reconsider those beliefs?

Do you see this as an adversity?   Why?

Do you see this as an opportunity?   Why?

When you start to review your plans, what is your baseline SUDS:

SUDS intensity (0–10)

How does this situation fit with what you had thought about before?   Why?

Does thinking about this change your SUDS?   Why?

Now, the what, where, and how:

Think about how you are holding yourself hostage.

What alternative conclusion(s) do you want?

How will you encourage it?

Think about how likely this option seems.

How does your formalizing your approach help?

After you review these perspectives, what is your resulting SUDS:

SUDS intensity (0–10)

Do you think you might have used any of our other skills?

Which ones?

Now let's think about whether all this helped:

Does writing the goal statement make the task clearer?

Does writing the goal statement make the task more manageable?

Does writing the steps needed make the task clearer?

Does writing the steps needed make the task more manageable?

Will checking off each step as it was completed be helpful?

Does this process make your impression of the event more compelling?

Can you think of anything you might change in this skill to make it more personally useful?

How about the future? Do you think you will be able to put your results to the test?

All advocacy is, at its core, an exercise in empathy.

— Samantha Power

PRACTICE EMPATHY

Again, one of the best ways we can really integrate a skill into our lives is to make it personal. To do this, we need to see the value of it in our lives. By examining empathy, critical thinking, and listening, specifically as they promote personal communication, we can gain more insight into the importance of empathy as a resiliency skill. However, given our individual differences, personal habits, and a good dose of reality, take a breather and consider when and how you might best incorporate the concept of empathy into your life.

Reflect: Think of a situation in your life right now where empathy would be of benefit to you and the people in your life. Do you think empathy might make it easier for you to reach out to others? Might it help you to understand when someone else reaches out to you? Consider using TAPPS collaborative groups to clarify this event.

Checklist for Practicing Empathy

Can you think of a situation where you might benefit from the empathy skill?

Thinking carefully, what did you see as the issue(s) and need(s) that had to be addressed?

Identify, as best you can, the dilemma you face:

    Do you have any fears about working with other people?

    Do you have any thoughts about the possible gains from such cooperation?

    What does this reveal about your beliefs?

    Should you reconsider those beliefs?

    Do you see this as an adversity?   Why?

    Do you see this as an opportunity?   Why?

When you start to review your plans, what is your baseline SUDS:

    SUDS intensity (0–10)

    How does this situation fit with what you had thought about before?   Why?

    Does thinking about this change your SUDS?   Why?

Now, the what, where, and how:

    Think about how you are holding yourself hostage.

    What alternative conclusion(s) do you want?

    How will you encourage it?

    Think about how likely this option seems.

    How does your formalizing your approach help?

After you review these perspectives, what is your resulting SUDS:

SUDS intensity (0–10)

Do you think you might have used any of our other skills?

    Which ones?

Now let's think about whether all this helped:

    Does writing the goal statement make the task clearer?

    Does writing the goal statement make the task more manageable?

    Does writing the steps needed make the task clearer?

    Does writing the steps needed make the task more manageable?

    Will checking off each step as it was completed be helpful?

    Does this process make your impression of the event more compelling?

Can you think of anything you might change in this skill to make it more personally useful?

How about the future? Do you think you will be able to put your results to the test?

And, digging a little deeper, consider the following:

- Are there ways that you could listen more attentively?

_____

_____

_____

_____

- Do you have preconceived ideas that cloud your thinking?

_____

_____

_____

_____

- How could you improve your communication style?

_____

_____

_____

_____

- After applying and practicing empathy, have you noticed an improvement in your ability to be a more effective communicator and critical thinker?

_____

_____

_____

_____

Courage is what it takes to stand up and speak.
Courage is also what it takes to sit down and listen.

— Winston Churchill

APPLY EMPATHY TO YOUR COMMUNITY

Establishing and maintaining a good support system is essential to effective resiliency as a source of strength and as an opportunity to offer support to others. What techniques might you use to introduce the concept of empathy and what would be your specific expectation of the outcome?

_____

_____

_____

_____

What are the implications of expanding this skill to a community? Consider the following discussion points:

■ Define the community where you are intending to apply the skill.

_____

_____

_____

_____

■ Why do you think this skill is appropriate for the particular community?

_____

_____

_____

_____

■ How do you see the skill being administered?

_____

_____

_____

_____

Checklist for Applying Empathy to Your Community

Can you think of a community situation where you might benefit from empathy?

Thinking carefully, what did you see as the issue(s) and need(s) that must be addressed?

Identify, as best you can, the dilemma you face:

Do you have any fears about working with other people?

Do you have any thoughts about the possible gains from such cooperation?

What does this reveal about your beliefs?

Should you reconsider those beliefs?

Do you see this as an adversity? Why?

Do you see this as an opportunity? Why?

When you start to review your plans, what is your baseline SUDS:

SUDS intensity (0–10)

How does this situation fit with what you had thought about before? Why?

Does thinking about this change your SUDS? Why?

Now, the what, where, and how:

Think about how they are holding themselves hostage.

What alternative conclusion(s) do they want?

How will you encourage it?

Think about how likely this option seems.

How does your formalizing your approach help?

After you review these perspectives, what is your resulting SUDS:

SUDS intensity (0–10)

Do you think you might use any of our other skills?

Which ones?

Now let's think about whether all this helped:

Does writing the goal statement make the task clearer?

Does writing the goal statement make the task more manageable?

Does writing the steps needed make the task clearer?

Does writing the steps needed make the task more manageable?

Is checking off each step as it was completed helpful?

Does this process make your impression of the event more compelling?

How do you think you'll do as a mentor?

Can you think of anything you might change in this skill to make it more personally useful?

How about the future? Do you think you will be able to put your results to the test?

If you haven't any charity in your heart,
you have the worst kind of heart trouble.

—Bob Hope

REMEMBERING EMPATHY

In review, a considerable portion of human communication is nonverbal in nature. This consists of body language, gestures, tone of voice, facial expressions, and eye contact. Therefore, to become effective communicators, we need to learn to take into account both verbal and nonverbal messages. If we do not take the time to develop communication skills to include empathy, we may send messages contrary to our intentions or misinterpret the messages of others.

We will all reach some or all of these points in our careers and we need to plan for that day. This must not be when we are in the midst of the storm, but before. Don't forget empathy and the associated skills that are a source of strength. These can save our lives.

Remember that everyone you meet is afraid of something,
loves something, and has lost something.

— H. Jackson Brown

NOTES

1   Haney, Debbie. "From sympathy to empathy: My journey from clinician to patient." *Radiologic Technology* 88, no. 1 (2016): 113-114.

2   Sinclair, Shane, Kate Beamer, Thomas F. Hack, Susan McClement, Shelley Raffin Bouchal, Harvey M. Chochinov, and Neil A. Hagen. "Sympathy, empathy, and compassion: A grounded theory study of palliative care patients' understandings, experiences, and preferences." *Palliative Medicine* 31, no. 5 (2016): 437-447.

3   Chismar, Douglas. "Empathy and sympathy: The important difference." *The Journal of Value Inquiry* 22, no. 4 (1988): 257-266.

4   Paul, Richard and Linda Elder. *Critical Thinking: Tools for Taking Charge of Your Professional and Personal Life*. Upper Saddle River, NJ: Pearson Education, 2013.

5   Kaya, Hülya, Emine Şenyuva, and Gönül Bodur. "Developing critical thinking disposition and emotional intelligence of nursing students: A longitudinal research." *Nurse Education Today* 48 (2017): 72-77.

6   Cottrell, Stella. *Critical Thinking Skills: Developing Effective Analysis and Argument*. Houndmills, Basingstroke, and Hampshire: Palgrave Macmillan, 2011.

7   Mangena, Agnes and Mary M. Chabeli. "Strategies to overcome obstacles in the facilitation of critical thinking in nursing education." *Nurse Education Today* 25, no. 4 (2005): 291-298.

8   Song, Eun Ju, Ya Ki Yang, and Sook Kyoung Park. "Effects on critical thinking disposition and empathy on cultural competency in nursing students." *Journal of Korean Academy of Psychiatric and Mental Health Nursing* 25, no. 4 (2016): 347-355.

9   Branch Jr, William T. "The ethics of caring and medical education." *Academic Medicine* 75, no. 2 (2000): 127-132.

10 Paul, Richard W. *Critical Thinking: What Every Person Needs to Survive in a Rapidly Changing World*. Santa Rosa, CA: Foundation for Critical Thinking, 1990, 17-36.

11 Haslam, Nick. "Humanising medical practice: the role of empathy." *Medical Journal of Australia* 187, no. 7 (2007): 381-382.

12 Dean, Sue, Maralyn Foureur, Chris Zaslawski, Toby Newton-John, Nickolas Yu, and Evangelos Pappas. "The effects of a structured mindfulness program on the development of empathy in healthcare students." *NursingPlus Open* 3 (2017): 1-5.

13 Mercer, Stewart W., Maria Higgins, Annemieke M. Bikker, Bridie Fitzpatrick, Alex McConnachie, Suzanne M. Lloyd, Paul Little, and Graham C. M. Watt. "General practitioners' empathy and health outcomes: A prospective observational study of consultations in areas of high and low deprivation." *Annals of Family Medicine* 14, no. 2 (2016): 117-124.

14 Hojat, Mohammadreza, Michael J. Vergare, Kaye Maxwell, George Brainard, Steven K. Herrine, Gerald A. Isenberg, Jon Veloski, and Joseph S. Gonnella. "The devil is in the third year: A longitudinal study of erosion of empathy in medical school." *Academic Medicine* 84, no. 9 (2009): 1182-1191.

15 Neumann, Melanie, Friedrich Edelhäuser, Diethard Tauschel, Martin R. Fischer, Markus Wirtz, Christiane Woopen, Aviad Haramati, and Christian Scheffer. "Empathy decline and its reasons: A systematic review of studies with medical students and residents." *Academic Medicine* 86, no. 8 (2011): 996-1009.

16 Raab, Kelley. "Mindfulness, self-compassion, and empathy among health care professionals: A review of the literature." *Journal of Health Care Chaplaincy* 20, no. 3 (2014): 95-108.

17 Benzo, Roberto P., Janae L. Kirsch, and Carlie Nelson. "Compassion, mindfulness and the happiness of health care workers." *Explore: The Journal of Science and Healing* 13, no. 3 (2017): 201-206.

18 Haramati, Aviad, Sian Cotton, Jamie S. Padmore, Hedy S. Wald, and Peggy A. Weissinger. "Strategies to promote resilience, empathy and well-being in the health professions: Insights from the 2015 CENTILE Conference." *Medical Teacher* 39, no. 2 (2017): 118-119.

19 Johnson, David W. *Reaching Out: Interpersonal Effectiveness and Self-Actualization* 8th ed. Boston: Allyn and Bacon, 2002.

20 Siebert, Darcy Clay. "Help seeking for AOD misuse among social workers: Patterns, barriers, and implications." *Social Work* 50, no. 1 (2005): 65-75.

21 Moll, Sandra E. "The web of silence: A qualitative case study of early intervention and support for healthcare workers with mental ill-health." *BMC Public Health* 14, no. 1 (2014): 138.

22 Kay, Margaret, Geoffrey Mitchell, Alexandra Clavarino, and Jenny Doust. "Doctors as patients: A systematic review of doctors' health access and the barriers they experience." *British Journal of General Practitioners* 58, no. 552 (2008): 501-508.

23 Donahue, Amy K. and Robert V. Tuohy. "Lessons we don't learn: A study of the lessons of disasters, why we repeat them, and how we can learn them." *Homeland Security Affairs* 2, no. 2 (2006).

24   Fuchs, Martin. "Reaching out; or, Nobody exists in one context only: Society as translation." *Translation Studies* 2, no. 1 (2009): 21-40.

25   Galdas, Paul M., Francine Cheater, and Paul Marshall. "Men and health help-seeking behaviour: Literature review." *Journal of Advanced Nursing* 49, no. 6 (2005): 616-623.

26   Allen, Christopher T., Rebecca Ridgeway, and Suzanne C. Swan. "College students' beliefs regarding help seeking for male and female sexual assault survivors: Even less support for male survivors." *Journal of Aggression, Maltreatment & Trauma* 24, no. 1 (2015): 102-115.

27   Juvrud, Joshua and Jennifer L. Rennels. "I don't need help: Gender differences in how gender stereotypes predict help-seeking." *Sex Roles* 76, no. 1-2 (2017): 27-39.

28   Steege, Linsey M. and Jessica G. Rainbow. "Fatigue in hospital nurses—'supernurse' culture is a barrier to addressing problems: A qualitative interview study." *International Journal of Nursing Studies* 67 (2017): 20-28.

29   Singer, Sara J., David M. Gaba, J. J. Geppert, Anna D. Sinaiko, Steven K. Howard, and K. C. Park. "The culture of safety: Results of an organization-wide survey in 15 California hospitals." *Quality and Safety in Health Care* 12, no. 2 (2003): 112-118.

30   Waters, Judith A. and William Ussery. "Police stress: History, contributing factors, symptoms, and interventions." *Policing: An International Journal of Police Strategies & Management* 30, no. 2 (2007): 169-188.

31   Sklar, David P. "Reaching out beyond the health care system to achieve a healthier nation." *Academic Medicine* 92, no. 3 (2017): 271-273.

32   van Dulmen, Sandra. "Person centered communication in healthcare: A matter of reaching out." *International Journal of Person Centered Medicine* 6, no. 1 (2016): 30-31.

33   Brown, C. Brené. *The Power of Vulnerability: Teachings on Authenticity, Connection, and Courage* [CD]. Louisville, CO: Sounds True, 2012.

34   Meyer, Frauke, Deidre M. Le Fevre, and Viviane M. J. Robinson. "How leaders communicate their vulnerability: Implications for trust building." *International Journal of Educational Management* 31, no. 2 (2017): 221-235.

35   Carter, Michele A. "Trust, power, and vulnerability: A discourse on helping in nursing." *Nursing Clinics of North America* 44, no. 4 (2009): 393-405.

36   Falcone, Rino and Cristiano Castelfranchi. "The socio-cognitive dynamics of trust: Does trust create trust?" In Falcone, Rino, Munindar Singh, and Yao-Hua Tan, eds. *Trust in Cyber-societies: Integrating the Human and Artificial Perspectives.* New York: Springer, 2001, 55-72.

37   Walter, Chris. [Book review] "Brown, Brené. (2015). "Daring greatly: How the courage to be vulnerable transforms the way we live, love, parent, and lead." *International Journal of Social Pedagogy* 5, no. 1 (2017): 180-183.

38   Cho, Ho Jin and Myun Sook Jung. "Effect of empathy, resilience, self-care on compassion fatigue in oncology nurses." *Journal of Korean Academy of Nursing Administration* 20, no. 4 (2014): 373-382.

39   Haramati, Aviad, Sian Cotton, Jamie S. Padmore, Hedy S. Wald, and Peggy A. Weissinger. "Strategies to promote resilience, empathy and well-being in the health professions: Insights from the 2015 CENTILE Conference." *Medical Teacher* 39, no. 2 (2017): 118-119.

40   Barker, Rhiannon, Jocelyn Cornwell, and Faye Gishen. "Introducing compassion into the education of health care professionals; Can Schwartz rounds help?" *Journal of Compassionate Health Care* 3, no. 1 (2016): 3.

41   Kelm, Zak, James Womer, Jennifer K. Walter, and Chris Feudtner. "Interventions to cultivate physician empathy: A systematic review." *BMC Medical Education* 14, no. 1 (2014): 219.

42   Shepherd, Katharine G., Colby T. Kervick, and Djenne-amal N. Morris. "Building capacity for collaboration." In *The Art of Collaboration: Lessons from Families of Children with Disabilities.* Rotterdam: Sense Publishers, 2017, 159-180.

43   Martins, Ana, Isabel Martins, and Orlando Pereira. "Challenges enhancing social and organizational performance." In de Pablos, Ordonez, Patricia and Robert D. Tennyson, eds. *Handbook of Research on Human Resources Strategies for the New Millennial Workforce.* Hershey, PA: IGI Global, 2017, 28-46.

44   Nicholl, Bill. "Empathy as an aspect of critical thought and action in design and technology." In Williams, P. John and Kay Stables, eds. *Critique in Design and Technology Education.* Singapore: Springer, 2017, 153-171.

45   Shiraev, Eric B. and David A. Levy. *Cross-cultural Psychology: Critical Thinking and Contemporary Applications.* New York: Routledge, 2015.

46   Andreou, Christos, Evridiki Papastavrou, and Anastasios Merkouris. "Learning styles and critical thinking relationship in baccalaureate nursing education: A systematic review." *Nurse Education Today* 34, no. 3 (2014): 362-371.

47 Paul, Richard W. *Critical Thinking: What Every Person Needs to Survive in a Rapidly Changing World.* Santa Rosa, CA: Foundation for Critical Thinking, 1990, 17-36.

48 Benard, Bonnie. *Resiliency: What We Have Learned.* San Francisco: WestEd, 2004, 7-42.

49 Brooks, Robert B. and Sam Goldstein. *The Power of Resilience: Achieving Balance, Confidence, and Personal Strength in Your Life.* New York: McGraw Hill, 2003, 125-182.

50 De Waal, Frans. *The Age of Empathy: Nature's Lessons for a Kinder Society.* New York: Three Rivers Press, 2009.

51 Arbilly, Michal and Kevin N. Laland. "The magnitude of innovation and its evolution in social animals." *Proceedings of the Royal Society B* 284, no. 1848 (2017): 284.

52 Zentall, Thomas R. and Bennet G. Galef Jr., eds. *Social Learning: Psychological and Biological Perspectives.* Madison, NY: Psychology Press, 2013.

53 Jenkins, Richard. *Social Identity*, 4th ed. New York: Routledge, 2014.

54 Sayer, Andrew. *Why Things Matter to People: Social Science, Values and Ethical Life.* Cambridge, New York: Cambridge University Press, 2011.

55 Burgoon, Judee K., Laura K. Guerrero, and Kory Floyd. *Nonverbal Communication.* New York: Routledge, 2016.

56 Remland, Martin S. *Nonverbal Communication in Everyday Life.* Los Angeles, London: SAGE Publications, 2016.

57 Tannen, Deborah. *You Just Don't Understand: Women and Men in Conversation.* New York: Quill, 2001, 23-74.

58 Coates, Jennifer. *Women, Men and Language: A Sociolinguistic Account of Gender Differences in Language.* New York: Routledge, 2015.

59 Farrell, Bill and Pam Farrell. *Men Are Like Waffles—Women Are Like Spaghetti.* Eugene, OR: Harvest House, 2016.

60 Headley, Jason. *It's Not About the Nail.* Republic Content, 2013. http://vimeo.com/66776386.

61 Cocksedge, Simon. "Learning to listen in primary care: Some educational challenges." *Education for Primary Care* 27, no. 6 (2016): 434-438.

62 Weyant, Ruth A., Lory Clukey, Melanie Roberts, and Ann Henderson. "Show your stuff and watch your tone: Nurses' caring behaviors." *American Journal of Critical Care* 26, no. 2 (2017): 111-117.

63 Nichols, Michael P. *The Lost Art of Listening: How Learning to Listen Can Improve Relationships.* New York: Guilford Press, 2009.

64 Markman, Howard J., Scott M. Stanley, and Susan L. Blumberg. *Fighting for Your Marriage: Positive Steps for Preventing Divorce and Preserving Lasting Love.* San Francisco: Jossey-Bass, 2001, 19-36.

65 Stone, Douglas, Bruce Patton, and Shiela Heen. *Difficult Conversations: How to Discuss What Matters Most.* New York: Penguin Books, 1999, 3-22.

66 Brooks, Robert and Sam Goldstein. *The Power of Resilience: Achieving Balance, Confidence, and Personal Strength in Your Life.* New York: McGraw-Hill, 2003, 99-124.

67 Miller, Rowland S. *Intimate Relationships.* New York: McGraw-Hill, 2014.

68 Tsen, Lawrence, Jo Shapiro, and Stanley Ashley. "Conflict resolution." In Kelz, Rachel R. and Sandra L. Wong, eds. *Surgical Quality Improvement.* Cham: Springer International Publishing, 2017, 75-83.

69 Alberti, Robert and Michael Emmons. *Your Perfect Right: Assertiveness and Equality in Your Life and Relationships.* Oakland, CA: New Harbinger Publications, 2017.

8

SOCIAL SUPPORT

Call it a clan, call it a network, call it a tribe, call it a family.
Whatever you call it, whoever you are, you need one.

— Jane Howard

OVERVIEW

Why: Social support is considered one of the best protections from suicide, PTSD, and the effects of stress.[1] Social support is the perceived and actual support provided through a supportive social network that will change throughout our lifespans.

How: To develop a system of social support we need to identify personal needs, individuals and the roles they play, and the contributions we make to sustain the system:

- Identifying perceived strengths and weaknesses aids in defining expected personal needs and desired people characteristics.

- When we identify the individuals in the support system, the roles they are to play, and how to contact them, we set our stage for functional support.

- Identifying the hoped-for personal contributions, those necessary to sustain the support system, provides opportunity for structural support.

Identifying a measure of change between before and after developing the goal and steps to meet the goal provides us a measure of our success. We use the Subjective Units of Distress Scale (SUDS) to help subjectively identify your stress level before, and again after, as somewhere between zero (0) and ten (10), where 0 corresponds to no stress and 10 to the highest level of stress you have ever experienced. The anticipation is that the SUDS level begins to decrease even after developing a goal statement and the steps to attain the goal. If your SUDS level increases, take some time to reassess the goal statement to assure it is attainable. And reassess the steps to assure that they have been adequately defined and there are a sufficient number. After all, you want to be able to check off each step and mark progress toward reaching your goal.

Goal Setting Skill—Social Support

Just as "It takes a village to raise a child," so does it take you helping others and welcoming their help in return.

Rate the stress level you perceive

Analog SUDS	Digital SUDS	Emoji SUDS
Actually, I'm not stressed	0	
A little stressed	1–3	
Somewhat stressed	4–6	
Quite a bit stressed	7–8	
It's really bad	9	
Run and hide!!	10	

Think about what's stressing you out. What might help?

Try and identify an objective to help you do that.

Write out a goal statement for your social support, about how you might look at your dilemmas differently, step-by-step.

Now get started! Don't be shy. Go for it!

Have you made any progress?

Rate the stress level you perceive now

Is it lower?

Yes	No
Congratulations!! You did it!! Now you can do this whenever you need it!	What might have gone wrong? Did you figure out all your steps? Did you actually do them all? Did you give yourself enough time? Was the time set aside to connect? Are you impatient and haven't allowed enough time to see change?

WHY SOCIAL SUPPORT?

*I am of the opinion that my life belongs to the whole community
and as long as I live, it is my privilege to do for it whatever I can.
I want to be thoroughly used up when I die,
for the harder I work the more I live.*

— George Bernard Shaw

We are herd animals and, as I mentioned earlier, the lone wolf is a Hollywood myth. Even heroes need mentors to be of service to others. A healthy support system or tribe is one in which we both give and receive. It is a two-way street. If all we do is offer support, we become exhausted. If all we do is take, we drain the resources of our network.

Thus, it is important in developing a healthy clan to identify personal needs, individuals, the roles they play, and the contributions each of us makes to sustaining the group. We all bring something to the table and the better we are able to recognize those strengths, within ourselves and others, the stronger our support system. Once again, the stronger our support system, the more protection we have from the effects of stress. A healthy support system is considered one of the best protections from suicide, PTSD, and the effects of stress.[2,3,4]

All of the skills we have been working on are tools to help nurture and maintain our clan during good times and times of stress.

> *This is so important I will repeat it one more time: one of the most significant factors in promoting resilient attitudes is the establishment and maintenance of a good support system.[5,6]*

Not only are social support systems a source of strength, but they also provide us opportunity to offer support and encouragement to others. Developing and acknowledging our strengths can help us become more self-efficacious, which means having the power to achieve a certain goal or the belief we are capable of achieving it.[7,8,9,10]

Some people may have significant roles in our social support system, while others may have more limited roles. We may have people who are supportive of our endeavors in the work setting but who have no contact with us outside of that setting. We may have people who can offer us advice about certain topics, for example, money or medical issues, but may not be able to offer us advice in other areas. It is important to remember that we may also play any of a variety of roles in other people's social systems. Taken alone, the contribution of a single individual to our social support system may not seem essential to our physiological and psychological well-being. Taken together, however, the contributions of all of the individuals who form our social support system are invaluable to our physiological and psychological well-being and the development of resilient attitudes.[11,12,13] Be aware too that we can develop focused support systems to better address specific needs, such as dealing with PTSD, burnout, and compassion fatigue.[14,15]

I don't know about you, but sometimes when I am overwhelmed I like to get away from it all and spend time alone. While there is merit to doing that, there is also a risk of making this the only coping strategy and not allowing the use of other resilience skills like reaching out.[16,17,18] This withdrawal into solitude, if unchecked, can become an avoidant behavior that risks social isolation and the breakdown of our support system. Remember that victims may see the dissolution of social support systems as inevitable, but survivors of trauma understand that there are concrete steps that they can take to build and strengthen their social support systems. The positive healing effect of support systems is particularly important for people who have survived horrific events.[19] Experts have observed that those of us who have at least one person whom we can call in the middle of the night to tell our troubles to go on to have better health than friendless people, and that those who isolate themselves when they are sick tend to get sicker.[20] The greatest risk to developing PTSD after a traumatic event is the lack of a social support system (fig. 8–1). And, in the context of resiliency, social support has demonstrated curative value following a traumatic event.[21,22] Don't forget we are social critters.[23,24]

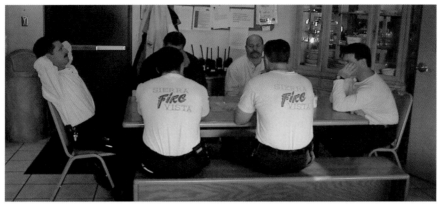

Fig. 8–1. Whether or not we acknowledge it, we are all social animals. (Courtesy of Mike Grill.)

THE HOW OF SOCIAL SUPPORT

Being deeply loved by someone gives you strength,
while loving someone deeply gives you courage.

— Lao Tzu

Because a healthy support system has two important functions—both to give and receive support—we'll need to explore what attitudes and behaviors we need from others and what it is about us that we have to offer to those in our support system. Put another way, what do we bring to the table? This latter aspect requires us look at our strengths or those characteristics that attract others to us. Taking compliments and acknowledging our strengths can be difficult for many of us. Have you ever given a compliment to someone or received one, only to hear or say, "I was just doing my job"? Where does this discounting of ourselves and our abilities come from? Culture, gender, personality styles, community, and family norms all influence how we acknowledge or dismiss our strengths and the feedback others give us about them.[25,26,27] As resilient people we are willing to confront these self-defeating patterns.

An exercise we frequently ask people to do is to take a piece of paper and write down three things they don't like about themselves. They're then asked how much time it took them to think of those three things. Unfortunately, most us can't write fast enough; that is because those flaws come to mind almost immediately. Try it:

_____

_____

_____

Next, we ask what three things they like about themselves. Inevitably this task takes longer than the three negatives. What are your three strengths?

_____

_____

_____

Focusing on personal strengths plays a vital role in developing a robust social support system. Identifying and acknowledging our strengths can help us become more self-efficacious and have a more positive self-image.[28,29] Again, self-efficacy is basically our belief in ourselves. Evidence-based research has clearly demonstrated a strong correlation between positive psychology and a vibrant support system.[30,31] Those of us that use positive self-talk and believe in ourselves are able to persist when faced with challenges, whether in academia, work, or our personal lives.[32,33,34] In other words, we are more resilient.

Another way to think of our social support system is as a resource that helps us to be resilient. Researchers have identified four types of resources that impact our resiliency: material resources, such as income; energy resources, such as availability of health insurance; work resources, such as a job; and interpersonal resources, such as social support.[35] A loss of any of these resources poses a challenge, increases stress, and decreases resiliency (fig. 8–2).

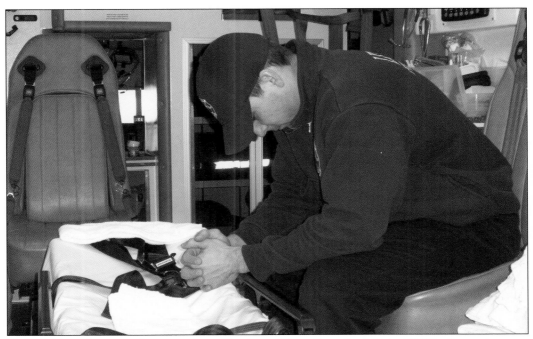

Fig. 8–2. A loss of resources increases stress. (Courtesy of Wayne Zygowicz, Littleton [CO] Fire Rescue.)

The other half of a healthy support system is an honest look at the people in our support system and what they bring to the table and what our needs are. Recognizing that we do have a need for others is important because the process helps us clarify our needs and select people who can best meet these needs. Sometimes, especially for those who are so focused on being of service to others, thinking about our needs and expressing them can be as difficult as acknowledging our strengths. This comes from negative beliefs about expressing those needs.[36,37]

Social Support Skill	
Identify support system quality (1–10)	
Quality:	?
Identify desired people characteristics	
Characteristics:	?
Identify people in system	
Spouse:	?
Children:	?
Siblings:	?
Best friends:	?
Coworkers:	?
Identify roles played by each person	
Spouse	?
Children:	?
Siblings:	?
Best friends:	?
Coworkers:	?
Identify personal strengths	
Like about myself:	?
Dislike about myself:	?
My contributions:	?
Identify goals	
Week 1:	?
Week 2:	?
Week 3:	?
Week 4:	?
Identify progress	
Week 1:	?
Week 2:	?
Week 3:	?
Week 4:	?
Identify potential improvements	
1:	?

2:	?
3:	?

Case study: Our lives can be complex. Say a colleague who has an 88-year-old Korean War veteran father declining with dementia reaches out to you. The family is struggling with decisions about the next level of care for their father, different perspectives from other family members, worries about their work, and the myriad activities of daily living. The colleague has a supportive spouse who picks up many of the latter duties and they have two adult children who live out of state but with whom they are in weekly contact. Your colleague is well known and respected professionally, but admits to feeling overwhelmed. The colleague confesses to being self-judgmental as well as judgmental toward others, and finds this worrisome.

You don't want to solve the problem for your colleague, but use the social support worksheet as a way to organize the information and thus empower the person in this difficult situation. Also think about the resiliency skills the colleague is already using.

It also gives you and your group an opportunity to familiarize yourselves with the worksheet (hint, hint!).

Example

Identify support system quality (1–10)

    Quality: 6

Identify desired people characteristics

    Characteristics: Honesty, insight

Identify people in system

Spouse:	Hera
Children:	Persephone, Prometheus, Cassandra
Siblings:	Poseidon, Hades
Best friends:	Medusa
Coworkers:	Bob, Carol, Ted, and Alice

Identify roles played by each person

Spouse:	Support and honest insight
Children:	Unconditional love and down-to-earth insight
Siblings:	Lifelong support and family insight
Best friends:	Unvarnished truth without regret
Coworkers:	Endeavor feedback and environmental insight

Identify personal strengths

Like about myself: Have ability to empathize. Solid work commitment and performance.

Dislike about myself: Can be judgmental. Don't have a sense of self-worth.

My contributions: I look to my strengths and recognize my personal likes and dislikes. I will bring both empathy and a strong sense of commitment.

Identify goals

 Week 1:   Re-examined my support system and better identified roles.

 Week 2:   Presented concept of perspective.

 Week 3:   Presented concept of goal setting.

 Week 4:   Discussed concept of mentorship.

Identify progress

 Week 1:   Discussed my contributions.

 Week 2:   Got some helpful feedback regarding time management.

 Week 3:   Got some feedback on the steps to meet my goal(s).

 Week 4:   Expressed desire for personal advancement.

Identify potential improvements

 1: Want to connect with spouse and children more often.

 2: Want to connect with best friend more often.

 3: Want to connect with someone who could be a mentor.

Social support is everything.

— Jordan Knight

FAMILY RESILIENCE

Sticks in a bundle are unbreakable.

— Kenyan proverb

Although we may have the odd relative who might distort our view of our family, when we think about our support system we typically include members of our family. And, in fact, family support or the lack of it can have a profound impact on us.[38,39,40] Acknowledging that there are stressful situations in life, that there are things that are difficult to bounce back from, can foster simple but effective coping skills. One simple thing we can do as parents to help our children become more resilient is read to them.[41,42] Studies indicate that one of the ways that we can increase our ability to empathize and develop critical thinking skills is by reading.[43]

The important thing to remember is that a healthy family support system is a place where we both give and receive. Too often, as parents, we are focused on what we can give our children to nurture them and increase their likelihood of success in life. In our fast-paced lives and our desire to provide our children with every opportunity, we create more stress for them and ourselves.[44,45]

We have talked about the importance of developing a routine (time management) for ourselves, and this is something we can model for our children as well as encourage them to create for themselves. The structure of a routine provides security, especially for younger children. However, today many parents feel that they have to keep the kids busy and so will have them scheduled for all the extracurricular activities they can cram into a day. Besides causing stress for the parents, it can also cause children to feel they have to perform and that whatever activity they are involved in is no longer fun.[46,47] What if we modeled and encouraged a little down time?[48] What if we as parents allowed our children or grandchildren to teach us the value of play?[49,50]

Research has shown that families are incredibly resilient, even in the face of adversity.[51,52,53,54] Think about the strengths of each of your immediate family members, even if they are young children. What and how do they contribute to your families' resilience?

_____

_____

_____

_____

While we usually think about family as biologically connected individuals, the family unit, especially for those in the first responder, medical, and the public service community, can be unique and sometimes even more intimate.[55,56] Military families, especially with multiple deployments, face severe stress that require great persistence, patience, and resilience.[56,57] For example, a resiliency workshop for children of military personnel at Ft. Belvior, Virginia, suggested to students that resiliency was like a muscle and the more they used the muscle the more it would help children be more resilient.[58] Interestingly, the workshop began by asking the students to identify "things that are difficult to bounce back from." Again, the point of this exercise was to acknowledge that there are stressful situations in life that we will confront and we need to have effective skills to deal with them. The workshop encouraged these five resiliency skills:

- Have a friend; be a friend.
- Take charge of your behavior.
- Set new goals and make plans to reach them.
- Look on the bright side.
- Believe in yourself.

Another thing that we can do with children when they are faced with stressful situations is to explore alternative ways of looking and thinking about the situation. Others suggest that when you are trying to evaluate a stressful situation, you make it a bit like a detective game (i.e., looking for the evidence for and against certain beliefs and attitudes).[59] The effort is intended to teach your children that they can find different perspectives.

In many situations, having a peer support system can also be beneficial to us. Certainly, peer support has been found to helpful across the health care provider spectrum.[60,61,62,63] These support systems typically revolve around work, but can include survivors of suicide loss, parents with infants in neonatal intensive care units, and veteran peer support, to name a few.[64,65,66] They can provide us a safe sanctuary. And, while they are beneficial and need to be an important part of our tool kit, we need to view them as just that—a part.

Resiliency throughout the ages

And in the end it is not the years of your life that count.
It is the life in your years.

— Abraham Lincoln

Another aspect of social support and resiliency is understanding that our system will evolve and change throughout our life spans.[67,68,69] We can be assured that our lives will change, sometimes for the better and sometimes for the worse, but most assuredly our lives will change. The question that arises is how we choose to deal with change (fig. 8–3). This is where our emotional intelligence can play a positive role.[70] Do we embrace change, dread change, or do we simply long for how things used to be? The attitude that we foster toward inevitable change is something that we can control.

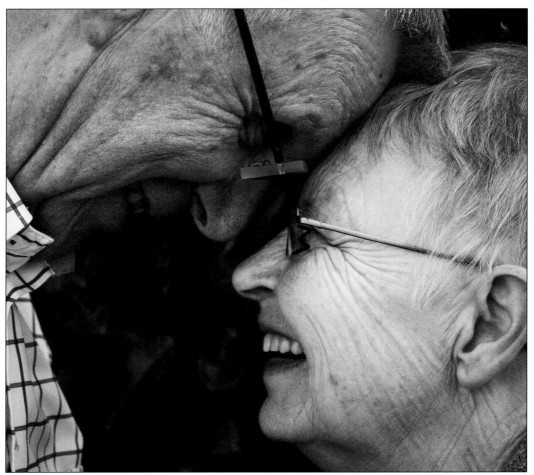

Fig. 8–3. How do you deal with life changes? (Courtesy of Lotte Meijer, unsplash.com.)

Understanding the stages of human development across the life span better prepares us to effectively cope with the stresses that challenge us as we continue to grow.[71,72,73,74,75] For example, older adults tend to use more avoidant-denial strategies in problem solving than do adolescents and younger adults.[76] Daniel Levinson, in his seminal model of human development across the life span, recognized two key concepts for each developmental stage to include a stable period and a transitional period.[77] The stable period is a time when a person makes crucial choices in life, builds a life structure around the choices, and seeks goals within the structure. The transitional period is the end of a stage and the beginning of a new stage. Each of these periods has inherent challenges. The transitional period has a significant amount of confusion and uncertainty, while the stability period has the stress of striving, particularly in the early phase. Think about your transition from childhood to adolescence as an example of this period of overlap. Who were your mentors and who did you mentor during times of transition (fig. 8–4)?

Mentorship

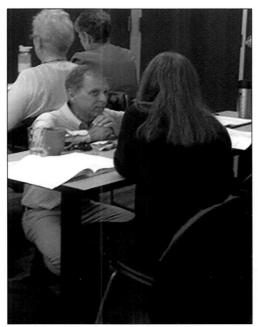

Fig. 8–4. Who was your mentor and who do you mentor today?

The delicate balance of mentoring someone is not creating them in your own image, but giving them the opportunity to create themselves.

— Steven Spielberg

Science confirms that those of us who have had mentors report having more satisfaction, career mobility/opportunity, recognition, and a higher promotion rate than nonmentored individuals.[78] Yet, mentorship can be complex for those unfamiliar with the process. Learners must make their own way and mentors must be prepared to face complex issues. Mentors must also understand that their efforts may not pay off quickly or perhaps ever.[79]

Mentoring is the belief that individuals may best learn through observing, doing, commenting, and questioning, rather than by simply listening.[80,81] As such, mentoring can be a process of educating an individual through the concept of a role model and can serve as an excellent tool for professional learning, both for the mentor and the person being mentored through systematic critical reflection. This reflection occurs by encouraging individuals to examine their practices and reappraise values, theories, and aspirations.

There are two types of mentoring: informal and formal or sponsored.[82] *Informal mentoring* is a relationship that occurs that is unplanned for the purpose of professional, personal, and psychological growth. Informal mentoring can be a meaningful qualitative experience. *Formal* or *sponsored mentoring*, on the other hand, is an intentional process that is typically the result of a planned mentoring program. Formal mentoring is designed to reach a variety of specific goals and purposes, defined by the setting in which the mentoring occurs.

The essence of mentoring is based on the idea of one-on-one teaching. The dynamics of mentorship typically include sharing control and creating opportunities for common learning. The mentorship may involve pursuing explorations, based on a learner's questions or understanding, into new areas. The learner is encouraged to develop the new skills necessary to work independently. Mentors try to model the very kind of learning they hope their learners will continue to pursue, the ideal of lifelong learning.[83] For example, Randy Pausch, a college professor, used a familiar lecture format to model his own life experiences into pragmatic lifelong learning lessons to be used by his children following his death from pancreatic cancer. *I highly recommend watching the video Randy Pausch—The Last Lecture Reprised, available on YouTube.*[84]

While we may not be mentoring in a formal manner within an educational setting, the phases of educational mentorship provide a good example of the change that does occur as a result of personal growth. This process can be considered as four phases.[85] The initial phase, typically occurring in the freshman year, is the period in which the relationship is formed through an organized process or through efforts to promote oneself through diligent work and opportunities for shadowing. The second phase, or cultivation phase, might occur during the sophomore and junior years, or even longer. During this phase, the positive expectations that emerged during the initiation phase are continually examined. The third phase, during or soon after a student's senior year, is a time when the learner experiences new independence and feelings of loss. The fourth phase is one of redefinition where both parties recognize that a shift in developmental tasks has occurred and that the previous mentorship process is no longer needed.

Mentoring can bring about immediate benefits for those engaged in these types of relationships, including increasing the student's likelihood of success.[86,87] It can also be a means for cultural change in the health care, public service, and education communities, where stress and its consequences are all too familiar.[88,89]

Reflection

How would you go about finding a mentor?

_____

_____

_____

_____

▪ How would you go about being a mentor?

_____

_____

_____

_____

> *If you are not spending ninety percent of your time teaching,*
> *you're not doing your job.*
>
> — Jim Senegal, CEO, Costco

INTERNALIZING SOCIAL SUPPORT

Life is not a solo act. It's a huge collaboration, and we all need to assemble
around us the people who care about us and support us in times of strife.

—Tim Gunn

As with all of the other skills we have worked on up to this point, think of a time in your life, in as much detail as possible, where you either gave or received support. Be aware of how old you were, what the situation was, and who the person was either needing or offering support. If you are health care provider who normally offers support, challenge yourself to think of a time when you reached out (fig. 8–5).

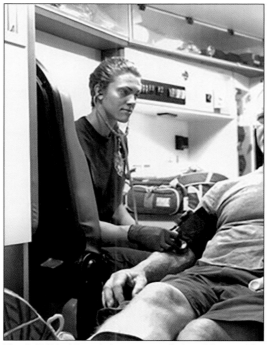

Fig. 8–5. Would you help someone find social support?

Checklist for Internalizing Social Support

Can you think of a situation where you benefited from the social support skill?

Thinking carefully, what did you see as the issue(s) and need(s) that had to be addressed?

Identify, as best you can, the dilemma:

What strengths did you call upon?

What weaknesses did you work to avoid?

Did you see this as an adversity?

Did you see this as an opportunity?

When you start to review this situation, what is your baseline SUDS?

SUDS intensity (0–10)

How did this situation fit with what you had thought about before?

Did thinking about this change your SUDS?

Identify the people who contributed to your system:

Spouse:

Children:

Siblings:

Best friends:

Coworkers:

Identify the roles played by each person:

Spouse:

Children:

Siblings:

Best friends:

Coworkers:

Identify the personal strengths on which you called:

Liked about myself:

Disliked about myself:

My intended contributions:

When you finish reviewing these circumstances, what is your resulting SUDS?

SUDS intensity (0–10)

Do you think you might have used any of our other skills?

Which ones?

Now let's think about whether all this helped:

Did writing the goal statement make the task clearer?

Did writing the goal statement make the task more manageable?

Did writing the steps needed make the task clearer?

Did writing the steps needed make the task more manageable?

Was checking off each step as it was completed helpful?

Did this process make your impression of the event more compelling?

Can you think of anything you might change in this skill to make it more personally useful?

How about the future? Do you think you will be able to put your results to the test?

Reflect: What made that experience memorable?

_____

_____

_____

_____

What was your motivation to use the concept of social support?

_____

_____

_____

_____

How were you able to achieve success with the concept of social support?

_____

_____

_____

_____

What did you learn about yourself and your support system?

_____

_____

_____

_____

Would you regard it as healthy, where you both give and receive support, or as out of balance? What can you do to change that?

_____

_____

_____

_____

When I do training events and we reach this point, I am reminded of my own professional career and the profound mentors I have had. I remember early in my career suffering a bit from the imposter syndrome, and reached out to an older physician. He allowed me to vent for a while and near the end of the conversation assured me, "The older you get, the one thing you know for sure is just how much you don't know everything."

EXTERNALIZE: APPLY SOCIAL SUPPORT AS A GROUP

True heroism is remarkably sober, very undramatic. It is not the urge to surpass all at whatever cost, but the urge to serve others at whatever cost.

— Arthur Ashe

Case Study: "You think it's going to be another 'feeling weak' complaint?" asks your partner.

"Could be, hard to be sure with an elderly patient," you respond.

It's early morning and you have been dispatched to an unknown medical incident. You recognize the address. You have been to this residence on several occasions. The chief complaint is typically something akin to feeling weak. You give the patient due diligence and perform a thorough examination, check the living conditions, and recommend transport for a more rigorous examination. The encounter always ends in a refusal for transport and your recommendation for follow-up with a physician.

"Well, if this ends up like the other calls we have had with him, would you be open to spending a few extra minutes there?" asks your partner.

You glance in the direction of your partner, anticipating a witty reply. Instead you respond, "Actually, I thought we might work with him on developing a social support network."

In your TAPPS groups, or individually, what might you offer as suggestions to these two paramedics?

Checklist for Externalizing Social Support

Can you think of a situation where you might benefit from the social support skill?

Thinking carefully, what do you see as the issue(s) and need(s) that have to be addressed?

Identify, as best you can, the dilemma:

> What strengths will you call upon?
>
> What weaknesses will you work to avoid?
>
> Do you see this as an adversity?
>
> Do you see this as an opportunity?

When you start to review this situation, what is your baseline SUDS?

> SUDS intensity (0–10)
>
> How does this situation fit with what you had thought about before?
>
> Does thinking about this change your SUDS?

Identify the people who contribute to your system:

Spouse:

Children:

Siblings:

Best friends:

Coworkers:

Identify the roles played by each person:

Spouse:

Children:

Siblings:

Best friends:

Coworkers:

Identify the personal strengths on which you called:

Like about myself:

Dislike about myself:

My intended contributions:

When you finish reviewing these circumstances, what is your resulting SUDS?

SUDS intensity (0–10)

Do you think you might have used any of our other skills?

Which ones?

Now let's think about whether all this helped:

Does writing the goal statement make the task clearer?

Does writing the goal statement make the task more manageable?

Does writing the steps needed make the task clearer?

Does writing the steps needed make the task more manageable?

Will checking off each step as it was completed be helpful?

Does this process make your impression of the event more compelling?

Can you think of anything you might change in this skill to make it more personally useful?

How about the future? Do you think you will be able to put your results to the test?

Reflect: What did you learn about yourself and your cohort in this exercise?

_____

_____

_____

_____

Can you see this application becoming useful in your work? How can you utilize the skill, both giving and receiving, more frequently?

_____

_____

_____

_____

The best way to find yourself is to lose yourself in the service of others.

— Mahatma Gandhi

PRACTICE SOCIAL SUPPORT

Think of a situation in your life right now where using the skill of social support might be of benefit to you.

It did not really matter what we expected from life,
but rather what life expected from us.

—Viktor Frankl

APPLY SOCIAL SUPPORT TO A COMMUNITY

Finally, you are asked to think about ways that you can apply this skill to strengthen your community, as you define it.

Just as people can be taught to be resilient, so can communities. The Substance Abuse and Mental Health Services Administration (SAMHSA) points out that *community resilience* is the ability of the individual and the collective community to respond to adversity and change.[90,91] Community resilience emerges as:

- Connectedness
- Commitment to community
- Shared values
- Structure, roles, and responsibilities that exist throughout the community
- Supportive
- Good communication
- Resource sharing
- Volunteerism
- Responsive organizations
- Strong schools

Given that the concept of social support requires effort to develop and sustain, what techniques might you use to introduce the concept of social support and what would be your specific expectation of the outcome?

One of the universal complaints of parents is that children do not listen to them. Most will agree, however, that children do watch, and that they model what they watch. For example, if children see parents viewing the world as an unsafe place, they can grow up to have the same world view. If children are repeatedly exposed to conflict, they can have trouble resolving problems with others. If children only get attention when they make mistakes, they may intentionally make mistakes because even negative attention may be valued more than no attention. Alternatively, if children see resilient attitudes and behaviors, they can model these.[91] If children see their parents accepting responsibility for their own behavior, they can as well. Children who demonstrate resiliency tend to have good cognitive ability and temperaments that facilitate good social relationships.[92]

By modeling engagement with our various communities and including our families in this process, we build character and citizenship through an educational approach known as *service-learning* (fig. 8–6).[93]

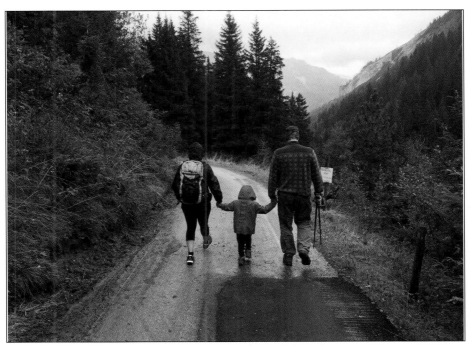

Fig. 8–6. Does your family keep rituals and traditions? (unsplash.com)

We can build upon existing elements of family strength to promote resiliency.[94] Consider, for example, the situation where a grandparent who has lost contact with his or her grandchildren can experience depressive symptoms for years.[95] Family members thus need to recognize the many ways that family members express their caring, such as by keeping open communication, maintaining and strengthening relationships, doing positive things for other family members, collaborating on problem solving, and managing conflicts.[96] Families are encouraged to develop and maintain rituals and traditions such as eating meals together and asking family members to share their accomplishments.

Checklist for Applying Social Support to Your Community

Can you think of a community situation that might benefit from the social support skill?

Thinking carefully, what do you see as the issue(s) and need(s) that have to be addressed?

Identify, as best you can, the dilemma:

What strengths might you call upon?

What weaknesses will you work to avoid?

Do you see this as an adversity?

Do you see this as an opportunity?

When you start to review this situation, what is your baseline SUDS?

SUDS intensity (0–10)

How does this situation fit with what you had thought about before?

Does thinking about this change your SUDS?

Identify people who might contribute to the current system:

Advocate 1:

Advocate 2:

Advocate 3:

Advocate 4:

Advocate 5:

Identify the roles played by each person:

Advocate 1:

Advocate 2:

Advocate 3:

Advocate 4:

Advocate 5:

Identify the personal strengths on which you will call:

Like about myself:

Dislike about myself:

My intended contributions:

When you finish reviewing these circumstances, what is your resulting SUDS?

SUDS intensity (0–10)

Do you think you might have used any of our other skills?

Which ones?

Now let's think about whether all this helped:

Does writing the goal statement make the task clearer?

Does writing the goal statement make the task more manageable?

Does writing the steps needed make the task clearer?

Does writing the steps needed make the task more manageable?

Will checking off each step as it was completed be helpful?

Does this process make your impression of the event more compelling?

How do you think you'll do as a mentor?

Can you think of anything you might change in this skill to make it more personally useful?

How about the future? Do you think you will be able to put your results to the test?

When you cease to make a contribution, you begin to die.

— Eleanor Roosevelt

REMEMBERING SOCIAL SUPPORT

Having a healthy support system, where we both give and receive support, is the most important resiliency skill. The skills we have explored have brought us to this point (fig. 8–7). What makes this skill memorable for you? Is it a celebration of the people you have surrounded yourself with? Is it the challenges you face in strengthening your existing support system? Is it the time when you needed a mentor and that someone was there for you? Is it the time when you were a mentor to someone?

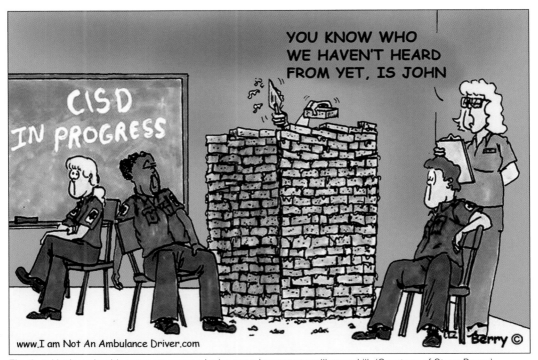

Fig. 8–7. Having a healthy support system is the most important resiliency skill. (Courtesy of Steve Berry.)

Among the many things I am reminded of about the importance of social support is the relationship between Forrest Gump and Lieutenant Dan in *Forrest Gump*. It is a reminder of the healing nature of social support. From the video, review the following chapters that illustrate this: Lieutenant Dan (00:40:38), Wounded in the Buttocks (00:56:31), Happy New Year (01:17:01), Bubba Gump (01:34:58), and Beloved Mother, Wife and Friend (02:04:46).

Summing up, my colleagues at the Mesa, Arizona, Fire Academy have a great exercise to remember the importance of this skill. They call it "Who ya gonna call?"

Who Ya Gonna Call?

When your water heater breaks, who ya gonna call?

Name: _____ Address: _____

Phone: _____ _____

email: _____ _____

When your car is having trouble, who ya gonna call?

Name: _____ Address: _____

Phone: _____ _____

email: _____ _____

When you've had a fight with your significant other, who ya gonna call?

Name: _____ Address: _____

Phone: _____ _____

email: _____ _____

When you've been having recurrent nightmares about your work, who ya gonna call?

Name: _____ Address: _____

Phone: _____ _____

email: _____ _____

When you've gone on a bunch of peds calls and you are flooded with intrusive memories, who ya gonna call?

Name: _____ Address: _____

Phone: _____ _____

email: _____ _____

When you're drinking too much to numb yourself out and you're thinking maybe everyone would be better off without you being around, who ya gonna call?

Name: _____ Address: _____

Phone: _____ _____

email: _____ _____

If you haven't, put these names, phone numbers, and other contact information in your cellphone. Do it before the fertilizer hits the ventilation system and before the crisis becomes overwhelming. Do it, understanding that the names may change over time.

The family. We were a strange little band of characters trudging through life sharing diseases and toothpaste, coveting one another's desserts, hiding shampoo, borrowing money, locking each other out of our rooms, inflicting pain and kissing to heal it in the same instant, loving, laughing, defending, and trying to figure out the common thread that bound us all together.

— Erma Bombeck

NOTES

1   Brewin, Chris R., Bernice Andrews, and John D. Valentine. "Meta-analysis of risk factors for posttraumatic stress disorder in trauma-exposed adults." *Journal of Consulting and Clinical Psychology* 68, no. 5 (2000): 748-766.

2   Cocking, Christopher. "Collective resilience and social support in the face of adversity: Evidence from social psychology." In Kumar, Updesh, ed. *Routledge International Handbook of Psychosocial Resilience.* London: Routledge, 2016, 111-123.

3   Wang, Lin, Hong Tao, Barbara J. Bowers, Roger Brown, and Yaqing Zhang. "Influence of social support and self-efficacy on resilience of early career registered nurses." *Western Journal of Nursing Research* (2017): DOI 0193945916685712.

4   Yu, Yongju, Li Peng, Long Chen, Ling Long, Wei He, Min Li, and Tao Wang. "Resilience and social support promote posttraumatic growth of women with infertility: The mediating role of positive coping." *Psychiatry Research* 215, no. 2 (2014): 401-405.

5   Zang, Yinyin, Thea Gallagher, Carmen P. McLean, Hallie S. Tannahill, Jeffrey S. Yarvis, Edna B. Foa, and STRONG STAR Consortium. "The impact of social support, unit cohesion, and trait resilience on PTSD in treatment-seeking military personnel with PTSD: The role of posttraumatic cognitions." *Journal of Psychiatric Research* 86 (2017): 18-25.

6   McSharry, Patsy and Fiona Timmins. "Promoting healthy lifestyle behaviours and well-being among nursing students." *Nursing Standard* 31, no. 24 (2017): 51-63.

7   Shoshani, Anat and Michelle Slone. "The resilience function of character strengths in the face of war and protracted conflict." *Frontiers in Psychology* 6 (2016).

8   Truebridge, Sara. *Resilience Begins with Beliefs: Building on Student Strengths for Success in School.* New York and London: Teachers College Press, 2014.

9   Leslie, Leigh A. and Sally A. Koblinsky. "Returning to civilian life: Family reintegration challenges and resilience of women veterans of the Iraq and Afghanistan wars." *Journal of Family Social Work* 20, no. 2 (2017): 106-123.

10 Bandura, Albert. *Self-Efficacy: The Exercise of Control.* New York: W. H. Freeman and Co., 1997.

11 Sarason, Irwin G., ed. *Social Support: Theory, Research and Applications* Vol. 24. Cham: Springer, 2013.

12 Uchino, Bert N. "Social support and health: A review of physiological processes potentially underlying links to disease outcomes." *Journal of Behavioral Medicine* 29, no. 4 (2006): 377-387.

13 Feeney, Brooke C. and Nancy L. Collins. "A new look at social support: A theoretical perspective on thriving through relationships." *Personality and Social Psychology Review* 19, no. 2 (2015): 113-147.

14 Repper, Julie and Tim Carter. "A review of the literature on peer support in mental health services." *Journal of Mental Health* 20, no. 4 (2011): 392-411.

15 Shapiro, Jo and Pamela Galowitz. "Peer support for clinicians: A programmatic approach." *Academic Medicine* 91, no. 9 (2016): 1200-1204.

16 Lay, Jennifer, C. Hoppmann, and A. Mahmood. "Aloneness need not be lonely: Varieties and predictors of positive solitude experiences in daily life." *European Health Psychologist* 18, no. S (2016): 1048.

17 Ren, Dongning. *Solitude Seeking: The Good, the Bad, and the Balance* [dissertation]. Purdue University, 2016.

18 Nouwen, Henri J. M. *Out of Solitude: Three Meditations on the Christian Life.* Notre Dame: IN: Ave Maria Press, 2004.

19 Bloom, Sandra L. "By the crowd they have been broken, by the crowd they shall be healed: The social transformation of trauma." In Tedeschi, Richard G., Crystal L. Park and Lawrence G. Calhoun, eds. *Posttraumatic Growth: Positive Change in the Aftermath of Crisis.* Mahwah, NJ: Lawrence Erlbaum Publishers, 1998, 173-208.

20 Seligman, Martin E. P. *Learned Optimism: How to Change Your Mind and Your Life.* New York: Random House, 2006, 174.

21   Koenen, Karestan C., Jeanne M. Stellman, Steven D. Stellman, and John F. Sommer Jr. "Risk factors for course of posttraumatic stress disorder among Vietnam veterans: A 14-year reflection of American Legionnaires." *Journal of Consulting and Clinical Psychology* 71, no. 6 (2003): 980-986.

22   Bonanno, George A., Sandro Galea, Angela Bucciarelli, and David Vlahov. "What predicts psychological resilience after disaster? The role of demographic, resources, and life stress." *Journal of Consulting and Clinical Psychology* 75, no. 5 (2007): 671-682.

23   Miller, Anna. "Friends wanted." *Monitor on Psychology* 45, no. 1 (2014): 54-58.

24   Cacioppo, John T. and William Patrick. *Loneliness: Human Nature and the Need for Social Connection.* New York: W.W. Norton & Co., 2011, 92-112.

25   Kille, David R., Richard P. Eibach, Joanne V. Wood, and John G. Holmes. "Who can't take a compliment? The role of construal level and self-esteem in accepting positive feedback from close others." *Journal of Experimental Social Psychology* 68 (2017): 40-49.

26   Tang, Chen-Hsin and Grace Qiao Zhang. "A contrastive study of compliment responses among Australian English and Mandarin Chinese speakers." *Journal of Pragmatics* 41, no. 2 (2009): 325-345.

27   Daikuhara, Midori. "A study of compliments from a cross-cultural perspective: Japanese vs. American English." *Working Papers in Educational Linguistics* (WPEL) 2, no. 2 (1986): 6.

28   Bandura, Albert. "Self-efficacy: Toward a unifying theory of behavior change." *Psychological Review* 84, no. 4 (1977): 191-215.

29   Alessandri, Guido, Laura Borgogni, Wilmar B. Schaufeli, Gian Vittorio Caprara, and Chiara Consiglio. "From positive orientation to job performance: The role of work engagement and self-efficacy beliefs." *Journal of Happiness Studies* 16, no. 3 (2015): 767-788.

30   O'Connell, Brenda H., Deirdre O'Shea, and Stephen Gallagher. "Enhancing social relationships through positive psychology activities: A randomised controlled trial." *Journal of Positive Psychology* 11, no. 2 (2016): 149-162.

31   Green, Suzy, Olivia Evans, and Belinda Williams. "Positive psychology at work: Research and practice." In *Positive Psychology Interventions in Practice.* Cham: Springer International Publishing, 2017, 185-206.

32   Marsh, Herbert W. and Marjorie Seaton. "Academic self-concept." In Hattie, John and Eric M. Anderman, eds. *International Guide to Student Achievement.* New York: Routledge, 2013, 62-63.

33   Blanchfield, Anthony William, James Hardy, Helma Majella De Morree, Walter Staiano, and Samuele Maria Marcora. "Talking yourself out of exhaustion: The effects of self-talk on endurance performance." *Medicine and Science in Sports Exerercise* 46, no. 5 (2014): 998-1007.

34   Horne, Rebecca M. and Matthew D. Johnson. "Gender role attitudes, relationship efficacy, and self-disclosure in intimate relationships." *Journal of Social Psychology* 158, no. 1 (2018): 37-50.

35   Bonanno, George A., Sandro Galea, Angela Bucciarelli, and David Vlahov. "Psychological resilience after disaster: New York City in the aftermath of the September 11th terrorist attack." *Psychological Science* 17, no. 3 (2006): 181-186.

36   Granek, Leeat, Merav Ben-David, Ora Nakash, Michal Cohen, Lisa Barbera, Samuel Ariad, and Monika K. Krzyzanowska. "Oncologists' negative attitudes towards expressing emotion over patient death and burnout." *Supportive Care in Cancer* 25, no. 5 (2017): 1607-1614.

37   Greene-Shortridge, Tiffany M., Thomas W. Britt, and Carl Andrew Castro. "The stigma of mental health problems in the military." *Military Medicine* 172, no. 2 (2007): 157-161.

38   Hawley, Dale R. and Laura DeHaan. "Toward a definition of family resilience: Integrating life-span and family perspectives." *Family Process* 35, no. 3 (1996): 283-298.

39   Farrell, Anne F., Gary L. Bowen, and Samantha A. Goodrich. "Strengthening family resilience." In Arditti, Joyce A., ed. *Family Problems: Stress, Risk, and Resilience.* Chichester, West Sussex: John Wiley & Sons, 2014, 273-288.

40   Borge, Anne I. H., Frosso Motti-Stefanidi, and Ann S. Masten. "Resilience in developing systems: The promise of integrated approaches for understanding and facilitating positive adaptation to adversity in individuals and their families." *European Journal of Developmental Psychology* 13, no. 3 (2016): 293-296.

41   Massaro, Dominic W. "Reading aloud to children: Benefits and implications for acquiring literacy before schooling begins." *American Journal of Psychology* 130, no. 1 (2017): 63-72.

42   Bjorklund, David F. and Kayla B. Causey. *Children's Thinking: Cognitive Development and Individual Differences.* Thousand Oaks, CA: SAGE Publications, 2017.

43   Li, Mengyi, P. Karen Murphy, Jianan Wang, Linda H. Mason, Carla M. Firetto, Liwei Wei, and Kyung Sun Chung. "Promoting reading comprehension and critical-analytic thinking: A comparison of three approaches with fourth and fifth graders." *Contemporary Educational Psychology* 46 (2016): 101-115.

44   Palmer, Sue. *Toxic Childhood: How the Modern World is Damaging Our Children and What We Can Do about It.* London: Orion, 2015.

45   Levine, Madeline. *The Price of Privilege: How Parental Pressure and Material Advantage Are Creating a Generation of Disconnected and Unhappy Kids.* New York: HarperCollins, 2006.

46   Masten, Ann S. and Amy R. Monn. "Child and family resilience: A call for integrated science, practice, and professional training." *Family Relations* 64, no. 1 (2015): 5-21.

47   Dacey, John S., Martha D. Mack, and Lisa B. Fiore. *Your Anxious Child: How Parents and Teachers Can Relieve Anxiety in Children*. Chichester, West Sussex: John Wiley & Sons, 2016.

48   Jay, Susan M. and Charles H. Elliott. "A stress inoculation program for parents whose children are undergoing painful medical procedures." *Journal of Consulting and Clinical Psychology* 58, no. 6 (1990): 799-804.

49   Else, Perry. *The Value of Play*. London: Bloomsbury Publishing, 2009.

50   O'Connor, Dee. "Loving learning: The value of play within contemporary primary school pedagogy." In Lynch, Sandra, Deborah Pike, and Cynthia Beckett. *Multidisciplinary Perspectives on Play from Birth and Beyond*. Singapore: Springer, 2017, 93-107.

51   Walsh, Froma. "Family resilience: Strengths forced through adversity." In Walsh, Froma, ed. *Normal Family Processes: Growing Diversity and Complexity*. New York: Guilford Press, 2003, 399-423.

52   Browne, Charlyn Harper. "The Strengthening Families Approach and Protective Factors Framework: A pathway to healthy development and well-being." In Shapiro, Cheri J. and Charlyn Harper Browne. *Innovative Approaches to Supporting Families of Young Children*. Cham: Springer International, 2016, 1-24.

53   Nerenberg, Laura Supkoff, and Abigail Gewirtz. "Promoting children's resilience by strengthening parenting practices in families under extreme stress." In Kumar, Updesh, ed. *Routledge International Handbook of Psychosocial Resilience*. London: Routledge, 2016, 369.

54   Masten, Ann S. "Resilience in children threatened by extreme adversity: Frameworks for research, practice, and translational synergy." *Development and Psychopathology* 23, no. 2 (2011): 493-506.

55   Torres, Victoria A., Samantha J. Synett, Michelle L. Pennington, Marc Kruse, Keith Sanford, and Suzy B. Gulliver. "The risks and rewards of marriage for fire fighters: A literature review with implications for EAP." *EASNA Research Notes* 5, no. 3 (2016): 1-13.

56   Lester, Patricia, Li-Jung Liang, Norweeta Milburn, Catherine Mogil, Kirsten Woodward, William Nash, Hilary Aralis, et al. "Evaluation of a family-centered preventive intervention for military families: Parent and child longitudinal outcomes." *Journal of the American Academy of Child & Adolescent Psychiatry* 55, no. 1 (2016): 14-24.

57   Piehler, Timothy F., Kadie Ausherbauer, Abigail Gewirtz, and Kate Gliske. "Improving child peer adjustment in military families through parent training: The mediational role of parental locus of control." *Journal of Early Adolescence* (2016): DOI 0272431616678990.

58   Kersting, Karen. "Resilience: The mental muscle everyone has." *Monitor on Psychology* 36, no. 4 (2005): 42.

59   Reivich, Karen and Andrew Shatté. *The Resilience Factor: 7 Keys to Finding Your Inner Strength and Overcoming Life's Inevitable Obstacles*. New York: Broadway Books, 2002, 252-281.

60   Witt, Katrina, Allison Milner, Amanda Allisey, Lauren Davenport, and Anthony D. LaMontagne. "Effectiveness of suicide prevention programs for emergency and protective services employees: A systematic review and meta-analysis." *American Journal of Industrial Medicine* 60, no. 4 (2017): 394-407.

61   Van Pelt, Frederick. "Peer support: Healthcare professionals supporting each other after adverse medical events." *Quality and Safety in Health Care* 17, no. 4 (2008): 249-252.

62   Hu, Yue-Yung, Megan L. Fix, Nathanael D. Hevelone, Stuart R. Lipsitz, Caprice C. Greenberg, Joel S. Weissman, and Jo Shapiro. "Physicians' needs in coping with emotional stressors: The case for peer support." *Archives of Surgery* 147, no. 3 (2012): 212-217.

63   Shapiro, Jo and Pamela Galowitz. "Peer support for clinicians: A programmatic approach." *Academic Medicine* 91, no. 9 (2016): 1200-1204.

64   SOSL, Survivors of Suicide Loss. https://www.soslsd.org/.

65   Hall, Sue L., D. J. Ryan, J. Beatty, and L. Grubbs. "Recommendations for peer-to-peer support for NICU parents." *Journal of Perinatology* 35, suppl. 1 (2015): S9-13.

66   U.S. Dept. Veterans Affairs. "PTSD: National Center for PTSD: Peer Support Groups." http://www.ptsd.va.gov/public/treatment/cope/peer_support_groups.asp.

67   Masten, Ann S. and Margaret O. Wright. "Resilience over the lifespan: Developmental perspectives on resistance, recovery, and transformation." In Reich, John W. and Alex J. Zautra, eds. *Handbook of Adult Resilience*. New York: Guilford Press (2009): 213-237.

68   Wrzus, Cornelia, Martha Hänel, Jenny Wagner, and Franz J. Neyer. "Social network changes and life events across the life span: A meta-analysis." *Psychological Bulletin* 139, no. 1 (2013): 53-80.

69   Cummings, E. Mark, Anita L. Greene, and Katherine H. Karraker, eds. *Life-span Developmental Psychology: Perspectives on Stress and Coping*. New York and London: Psychology Press, 2014.

70   Chen, Yiwei, Yisheng Peng, and Ping Fang. "Emotional intelligence mediates the relationship between age and subjective well-being." *International Journal of Aging and Human Development* 83, no. 2 (2016): 91-107.

71   Lamont, Ruth A., Sharon M. Nelis, Catherine Quinn, and Linda Clare. "Social support and attitudes to aging in later life." *International Journal of Aging and Human Development* 84, no. 2 (2017): 109-125.

72   Reimers, Stian and Elizabeth A. Maylor. "Task switching across the life span: Effects of age on general and specific switch costs." *Developmental Psychology* 41, no. 4 (2005): 661-671.

73   Cavanaugh, John C. and Fredda Blanchard-Fields. *Adult Development and Aging.* Belmont, CA: Wadsworth, 2011, 531-550.

74   Horhota, Michelle, Andrew Mienaltowski, and Yiwei Chen. "Causal attributions across the adult lifespan." In Verhaeghen, Paul and Christopher Hertzog, eds. *The Oxford Handbook of Emotion, Social Cognition, and Problem Solving in Adulthood.* New York: Oxford University Press, 2014, 288-301.

75   Dikkers, Josje, Annet De Lange, and Beatrice Van der Heijden. "An integrative psychological perspective on (successful) ageing at work." In Parry, Emma and Jean McCarthy, eds. *The Palgrave Handbook of Age Diversity and Work.* London: Palgrave Macmillan, 2017, 67-88.

76   Southwick, Steven M., Brett T. Litz, Dennis Charney, and Matthew J. Friedman, eds. *Resilience and Mental Health: Challenges Across the Lifespan.* New York: Cambridge University Press, 2011.

77   Levinson, Daniel Jacob. *The Seasons of a Man's Life.* New York: Ballantine Books, 1978.

78   Fagenson, Ellen A. "The mentor advantage: Perceived career/job experiences of proteges versus non-proteges." *Journal of Organizational Behavior* 10, no. 4 (1989): 309-320.

79   Crutcher, Betty N. "Mentoring across cultures." *Academe* 93 no. 4 (2007): 44-48.

80   Nicholls, Gill. "Mentoring: The art of teaching and learning." In Jarvis, Peter, ed. *The Theory and Practice of Teaching.* Sterling, VA: Stylus Publishing, 2002, 157-168.

81   Palmer, Parker J. *The Courage to Teach: Exploring the Inner Landscape of a Teacher's Life.* San Francisco: Jossey-Bass, 2007, 191-224.

82   Galbraith, Michael W. "Mentoring toward self-directedness." *Adult Learning* 14, no. 4 (2003).

83   Chen, James R., Michael V. Fortunato, Alan Mandell, Susan Oaks, and Duncan RyanMann, "Reconceptualizing the faculty role: Alternative models." In Smith, Barbara L. and John McCann, eds. *Reinventing Ourselves, Interdisciplinary Education, Collaborative Learning, and Experimentation in Higher Education.* Boston: Anker Publishing, 2001, 328-339.

84   *Randy Pausch—The Last Lecture Reprised.* https://www.youtube.com/watch?v=ji5_MqicxSo.

85   Galbraith, Michael W. and Patricia Maslin-Ostrowski. "The mentor: Facilitating out-of-class cognitive and affective growth." In Bess, James L. and Associates. *Teaching Alone Teaching Together: Transforming the Structure of Teams for Teaching.* San Francisco: Jossey-Bass, 2000, 133-150.

86   Marshall, Jenna H., Edith C. Lawrence, Joanna Lee Williams, and James Peugh. "Mentoring as service-learning: The relationship between perceived peer support and outcomes for college women mentors." *Studies in Educational Evaluation* 47 (2015): 38-46.

87   Zammit, Katina, Margaret Vickers, Evelyn Hibbert, and Clare Power. "Equity buddies: Building communities of practice to support the transition and retention of students through their first year at university." In McDonald, Jacquie and Aileen Cater-Steel, eds. *Implementing Communities of Practice in Higher Education: Dreamers and Schemers.* Singapore: Springer, 2017, 373-394.

88   Henderson, Sarah N., Vincent B. Van Hasselt, Todd J. LeDuc, and Judy Couwels. "Firefighter suicide: Understanding cultural challenges for mental health professionals." *Professional Psychology: Research and Practice* 47, no. 3 (2016): 224-230.

89   Fisher, Edwin B., Muchieh Maggy Coufal, Humberto Parada, Jennifer B. Robinette, Patrick Y. Tang, Diana M. Urlaub, Claudia Castillo, et al. "Peer support in health care and prevention: Cultural, organizational, and dissemination issues." *Annual Review of Public Health* 35 (2014): 363-383.

90   Substance Abuse and Mental Health Services Administration (SAMHSA). "Resilience and Stress Management." https://www.samhsa.gov/dbhis-collections/resilience-stress-management.

91   MacDermid, Shelly M., Rita Samper, Rona Schwarz, Jacob Nishida, and Dan Nyaronga. *Understanding and Promoting Resilience in Military Families.* West Lafayette, IN: Military Family Research Institute, Purdue University, 2008.

92   Condly, Steven J. "Resilience in children: A review of literature with implications for education." *Urban Education*, 41 no. 3 (2006): 211-236.

93   D'Rozario, Vilma, Soo-Yin Tan, and Ava Patricia C. Avila. "Building character and citizenship through service learning." In Tan, Oon-Seng, Woon-Chia Liu, and Ee-Ling Low, eds. *Teacher Education in the 21st Century: Singapore's Evolution and Innovation.* Singapore: Springer, 2017, 233-252.

94   Benson, Peter L., Marc Mannes, Karen Pittman, and Thaddeus Ferber. "Youth development, developmental assets, and public policy." In Lerner, Richard M. and Laurence Steinberg, eds. *Handbook of Adolescent Psychology*, 2nd ed. Hoboken, NJ: John Wiley & Sons, 2004, 781-814.

95   Drew, Linda M. and Merril Silberstein. "Grandparents' psychological well-being after loss of contact with their grandchildren." *Journal of Family Psychology* 21, no. 3 (2007): 372-379.

96   Cole, Kelly A., James A. Clark, and Sara Gable. "Promoting family strengths." In Henderson, Nan, ed. *Resiliency in Action: Practical Ideas for Overcoming Risks and Building Strengths in Youth, Families, and Communities.* Ojai, CA: Resiliency in Action Press, 2007, 199-201.

FINAL THOUGHTS

*What we call the beginning is often the end. And to make an end
is to make a beginning. The end is where we start from.*

—T.S. Elliot

As you may have already guessed, this is not the end of your journey but the beginning. With practice, the skills we have explored will become a habit and these will ultimately shape your character and destiny. To truly bounce back from the stresses and difficulties that will confront us is to understand that the skills required to be resilient involve practice and flexibility.

While I believe that practice makes perfect, I also hold that "progress not perfection" is a good mind-set to have. Practicing the skills will not only make us better at them, but will allow us to explore other ways and places to use them. And thus, we all contribute to the evolution of this program. Fire, police, and EMS academies, the University of Arizona College of Nursing, and the Colorado Department of Emergency Preparedness have integrated these resilience skills into their educational curricula. Their contributions continue to clarify how best to disseminate and assimilate these skills into the care provider community.

I would encourage you to focus on where you have made progress in integrating these skills and use that information to inspire you to move forward. Yes, you will fail, which is a good thing. If viewed correctly, it can motivate you to greater resolve and have that learning be seen as an opportunity to correct your course.

One of the important reminders for me in this work is that the traumas people face do not occur in a vacuum. The first responders who come home after a horrific shift hoping to spare their family by being stoic and silent do not do themselves or their family any favors. My colleagues and I believe that to sustain resilient people we must have resilient families. Share the practice of these skills with your families.

Dr. Callahan, myself, and other contributors are working on new methods for learning these resilience skills, such as gamification. The hope is that you, your children, and your support system can use the story-telling skills involved in these gamified learning processes to find greater understanding of these and other resilience skills, and how they can be of benefit. For further information, you can contact them at http://www.onetreelearning.org/.

Our work continues to evolve as we develop and refine both the content and methods of delivery. We welcome your lessons learned, because this is how we all learn together.

M M

Act as if what you do makes a difference. It does.

—William James

INDEX